Sacroiliac Joint Dysfunction and Piriformis Syndrome

The Complete Guide for Physical Therapists

Paula Clayton

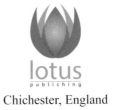

lotus
publishing

Chichester, England

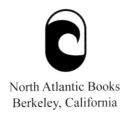

North Atlantic Books
Berkeley, California

First published in 2016 by
Lotus Publishing
Apple Tree Cottage, Inlands Road, Nutbourne, Chichester, PO18 8RJ, and
North Atlantic Books
PO Box 12327
Berkeley, California 94712

Anatomical Drawings Amanda Williams
Photographs Liz Vanegas de Quickenden
Photograph Overlays Emily Evans
Exercise Drawings Matt Lambert
Text Design Emily Evans
Cover Design Wendy Craig
Printed and Bound in the UK by Short Run Press Limited

Sacroiliac Joint Dysfunction and Piriformis Syndrome: The Complete Guide for Physical Therapists is sponsored and published by the Society for the Study of Native Arts and Sciences (dba North Atlantic Books), an educational nonprofit based in Berkeley, California, that collaborates with partners to develop cross-cultural perspectives; nurture holistic views of art, science, the humanities, and healing; and seed personal and global transformation by publishing work on the relationship of body, spirit, and nature.

North Atlantic Books' publications are available through most bookstores.
For further information, visit our website at www.northatlanticbooks.com or call 800-733-3000.

Disclaimer

Every effort has been made to include the most accurate and up-to-date information in this publication. However, the authors would be grateful for any errors to be brought to their attention. Neither the authors nor the publishers can take responsibility for misuse of this information or for injury caused by inappropriately applied treatment. Please consult a healthcare professional before applying any of the methods discussed in this text.

The publisher has made every effort to trace holders of copyright in original material and to seek permission for its use in *Sacroiliac Joint Dysfunction and Piriformis Syndrome*. Should this have proved impossible, copyright holders are asked to contact the publisher so that suitable acknowledgment can be made at the first opportunity.

British Library Cataloguing-in-Publication Data
A CIP record for this book is available from the British Library
ISBN 978 1 905367 64 1 (Lotus Publishing)
ISBN 978 1 623170 85 1 (North Atlantic Books)

Library of Congress Cataloging-in-Publication Data
Names: Clayton, Paula, 1966- , author. | Society for the Study of Native Arts
  and Sciences, sponsoring body.
Title: Sacroiliac joint dysfunction and piriformis syndrome : the complete guide for
  physical therapists / Paula Clayton.
Other titles: Sacroiliac joint dysfunction and piriformis syndrome
Description: Berkeley, California : North Atlantic Books, [2016] | Includes
  bibliographical references and index.
Identifiers: LCCN 2015045774 (print) | LCCN 2015046521 (ebook) | ISBN
  9781623170851 (pbk.) | ISBN 9781623170868 (ebook)
Subjects: | MESH: Physical Therapy Modalities—Handbooks. | Piriformis Muscle
  Syndrome—Handbooks. | Sacroiliac Joint—Handbooks.
Classification: LCC RD549.5 (print) | LCC RD549.5 (ebook) | NLM WE 39 | DDC
  617.5/81—dc23
LC record available at http://lccn.loc.gov/2015045774

Contents

Foreword by Dr. Gerry Ramogida

Applications for soft-tissue therapy have increased significantly over the last decade. Perhaps the greatest area of growth has been around sports and caring for athletes. Multiple soft-tissue manipulative (active-release techniques, soft-tissue release, myofascial release) and needling (including acupuncture, intramuscular stimulation, and dry needling) techniques have become mainstream tools in the therapist's "toolbox," whether to aid in athlete recovery, performance enhancement, or injury prevention.

This growth in soft-tissue therapy should come as no surprise given the influence soft-tissue health has in dictating athlete success. Perhaps this is because the soft tissues house many of the sensory organs and systems (Golgi tendon organs, muscle spindles, and capsular mechanoreceptors to name a few) that the central nervous system is dependent upon for coordinating the movements and producing the forces required for the specific demands of any given skill or action.

If the soft tissues do not move, stretch, contract, and "sense" optimally, we should not then expect optimal motor control, coordination, and output, and thus should not expect optimal performance. The best rehab programs cannot compensate for poor soft-tissue quality, as healthy soft tissue is required for optimal motor-unit activation and force production. We know through the work of individuals such as Carla and Antonio Stecco, Tom Meyers, and H. van der Wall that functional chains of agonists, synergists, antagonist muscles, and myofascial groups are directly connected via retinacula, intermuscular septa, interosseous membranes, and myofascial expansions. In fact, the Steccos' research has shown that over 40% of the musculotendinous tissue from muscle doesn't end at the bony insertion but blends into the previously mentioned soft-tissue structures. Given these facts, accurate assessment and diagnosis, and then choice of appropriate soft-tissue treatment intervention, are of paramount importance in meeting the needs of our athletes in the sporting environment.

Paula Clayton has been working in the performance arena for her entire career, first as a soft-tissue therapist and more recently as a physiotherapist. Given her accomplishments as a soft-tissue therapist (a mainstay for British Athletics, aiding in many athletes reaching Olympic and World-Championship podiums, along with years of involvement in Premiership soccer and rugby), I was surprised when she returned to school to become a chartered physiotherapist. If I had dedicated as much of my time and effort as Paula had to gaining unquestionable skill over many years, and helped so many reach the pinnacles of their respective sports, I couldn't imagine taking on a new full-time academic challenge. However, as Paula always has, she took this on and excelled. Given her extensive academic knowledge and unparalleled experience, this book brings together everything a therapist needs when working in the sports environment.

Sacroiliac Joint Dysfunction and Piriformis Syndrome: The Complete Guide for Physical Therapists offers the "how," but, more importantly, the "why," as to the map of approach one can take. I often say when teaching: if you cannot answer the *why* when beginning treatment, you shouldn't really do anything until you have an answer.

Having worked side by side with Paula at British Athletics for the three years leading up to the London 2012 Summer Olympic Games, where collectively our assembled team saw a decrease in injury frequency from in the 30% range (proportion of athletes unavailable for competition at any given time owing to injury) to single digits. This drop was almost as impressive as the team's steadily rising medal totals through the major competitions in those three years leading up to and through the games. These results did not occur by accident. Much of it was due to the hard work and expertise brought to British Athletics through individuals like Paula.

I invite you to use this book as a guide to help you improve your skills, and ultimately assist you in becoming a better therapist. The more skilled we become, the better our outcomes, the more likely given the right opportunity that our skills will have a small part in assisting athletes fulfill their aspirations, whether that be within a community-based team or as part of a federation at an Olympic Games. Sit back and be open to learning from someone who has repeatedly assisted athletes accomplish great things, for true success does not happen once but is sustained and repeated—that is the true mark of mastery. Paula Clayton has accomplished this type of mastery.

Dr. Gerry Ramogida is an internationally recognized chiropractor and performance therapist who has served on many Canadian national teams. He was the British Athletics "Lead" Performance Therapist for the 2012 London Olympics. Dr. Ramogida is currently working at Fortius Sport and Health in Vancouver, BC, as the Director of Chiropractic Services as well as serving as the medical director to the World Athletics Center (WAC) and WAC Canada.

Foreword by Neil Black

Having worked very closely with Paula over an eleven-year period (from 2003) within the English Institute of Sport (EIS) and British Athletics, I have found that rarely do you come across a practitioner who has such a clear understanding and total respect for all the members of the multidisciplinary team. Paula has a very unique skill set, including the very rare skill of having the understanding and confidence to know when to do nothing. She demonstrates highly accomplished assessment and evaluation skills, allowing her to make a strong contribution to the working diagnoses and treatment plans. She has a real understanding of functional and event-specific technical movement patterns, thereby allowing her to make an all-round contribution to performance enhancement. As a model professional, Paula is hugely respected by her colleagues in the multidisciplinary team and by coaches and athletes; she is massively valued for her personal and professional skills, commitment, and honesty, as well as for her listening and being supportive at all times. Paula has been a key member of the medical team attending most senior camps and competitions over the last three Olympic cycles (including Olympic and World Championships), making huge overall and individual contributions at all levels.

Many books currently on the market demonstrate single techniques, but Paula has endeavored to share all the "tools in her box" that can be used to address injury, dysfunction, and recovery. With careful use of current literature and detailed descriptions of assessment and treatment techniques, this book will become the one to buy for students, the newly qualified, and seasoned practitioners alike.

The reader of this book will be in the position to be fully informed, confident in the knowledge that not only are the techniques described here clinically relevant and effective but that their fundamental principles are supported by current research. Picking up this book today will have you well on the way to being able to deliver performance-impacting results with physical therapy techniques, both for the general public and for the athletic population.

Neil Black is the Performance Director at British Athletics. He was previously British Athletics' Chief Physiotherapist from November 2004, and Sports Medicine and Science Lead since December 2007. Neil has worked with the British national governing body and athletes attending most championships since the 1992 Paralympic Games.

Preface

Thank you for allowing me the privilege of sharing this book with you. I have tried hard to include everything that I think you will need to achieve a successful outcome, without, hopefully, being too exhaustive. I am passionate about helping people and about using soft-tissue techniques to get the results both I and my athletes and private patients are looking for, and to target the goals we have agreed during the assessment process.

I have been working in the field of performance-impacting soft-tissue therapy for many years, including four years in Premiership and Championship soccer and almost twelve years as a senior performance therapist with the English Institute of Sport and British Athletics. During this time I have had the incredible opportunity of travelling the globe with British Diving to a Commonwealth Games, and with British Athletics to three Olympic Games (Athens, Beijing, London) and countless World and European Championships as part of the GB track and field medical team.

Alongside my elite sport involvement, I have been running a very successful sports injury practice in the heart of Cleobury Mortimer in Shropshire with my husband Rick. I ran another in Birmingham University from 2013 to 2015 (which was recently relocated to Worcestershire), and I have just added a new practice in Harrogate.

I have taught on two sports therapy degree programs, delivered sessions to MSc students, and written a number of journal articles.

I have numerous soft-tissue-therapy qualifications in addition to a Football Association (FA) Diploma in the Treatment and Management of Injuries, an MSc in Sports Injury Management, and an MSc in Physiotherapy. I also deliver soft-tissue master classes to senior physiotherapists and soft-tissue therapists within Premiership and Championship soccer clubs and national governing bodies, and to soft-tissue therapists nationally and internationally through my company www.stt4performance.com.

I have level-five (Gold) membership with the Sports Massage Association (SMA; the association for soft-tissue therapists), for whom I am also a director and board member. I am a member of the Chartered Society of Physiotherapy, the Health Care Professions Council, and the Association of Chartered Physiotherapists in Sports and Exercise Medicine.

Whilst working, I have regularly been approached and asked if I would be prepared to teach the techniques I use. So, I developed a number of courses, and these are now delivered through my company STT4Performance. The courses are for therapists within sporting national governing bodies (NGBs), within soccer (including the UK Premier League), and to qualified therapists nationally. I was also asked if I would be interested in writing a book with step-by-step instructions covering the techniques that were introduced—so here it is. It's taken a long time to get to this point for lots of different reasons, but I am so proud to have finally put together a "one-stop shop" book. I hope that you begin to see results from the very first technique to the last.

I will regularly refer to the "athlete" when detailing assessments, therapy techniques, and processes within the following pages, but these techniques are also incredibly effective when working with the general public.

I have endeavored to cite relevant research for those therapists who strive for evidence-based practice; however, I would like to share the following quote with you:

> "External clinical evidence can inform, but can never replace, individual expertise, and it is this expertise that decides whether the external evidence applies to the patient at all and, if so, how it should be integrated into a clinical decision."
> (Sackett et al., 1996)

Whilst much progress has been made and lives have been saved through the systematic collation, synthesis, and application of high-quality empirical evidence, there have recently been signs that the focus of clinical care has shifted insidiously from the patient to the population subgroup, and that the "evidence-based tail has been wagging the clinical dog" (Greenhalgh et al., 2014).

Real evidence-based medicine has the care of the individual patients as its top priority, asking, "What is the best course of action for this patient, in these circumstances, at this point in their illness or condition?" (Huntley et al., 2012; Greenhalgh et al., 2014).

Talented individual therapists always have the potential to transcend the limitations of a particular kind of treatment. It's the skill of the therapist not the therapy technique itself that gets the results.

My hope is that this book in some way helps you to help others and that you find the techniques fit into your daily practice. Please remember that these techniques have evolved through years and years of trying and testing until results became the norm. However, they are only techniques—it's imperative that your anatomical and functional knowledge is able to support the techniques you are about to use and that you are continually assessing, adding the intervention, and reassessing, so that you have some outcome measures to enable you to reproduce a successful technique or adapt a not-so-successful technique.

I have unlimited respect for the fascial researchers of today and you will see I am strongly influenced by the works of Andry Vleeming, Robert Schleip, Carla Stecco, and Tom Myers, amongst others.

Before moving forward with the treatment suggestions contained within this book, please take a moment to really think about what is happening in the body when a structure is so dysfunctional that is it causing pain and an altered range of movement or gait, and remind yourself how the body adapts to this dysfunction by spreading the load and causing further dysfunction/pain. Ask yourself the question, "How did the SIJ or piriformis become like this?" Was it a primary or secondary adaptation following something like a biomechanical abnormality, a recent increase in training with altered gait, a recent ankle sprain, pelvic or lower back pain, shoulder or thoracic dysfunction, etc.?

Soft-tissue techniques vary from therapist to therapist. The ones that I am about to share with you are the ones I find are most effective. I would not presume to attempt to belittle or put aside other techniques, or encourage you to change your current practice; these are simply introduced as additional tools for your ever-growing toolbox—ideas that you may want to consider if you are not getting the results you require.

How to Use This Book

1. All of the tinted boxes contain additional information such as detailed anatomy or research facts. Whilst it's not imperative that these sections are read, I would strongly advise you to sit with a cup of coffee one day and read them, as they contain information that may answer some of your burning questions.

2. Prior to all treatments please ensure you have undertaken a thorough assessment:
   - Include red and yellow Flags in your subjective assessments.
     - Red (indicating more serious pathology)
       - (1) Constant unremitting pain
       - (2) Night pain
       - (3) Sudden and unexplained weight loss
       - (4) THREADOC[1]
     - Yellow (psychosocial)
   - Use your clinical reasoning to decide what action needs to be taken.
   - From the assessment, choose an outcome measure.
   - Implement your treatment or treatments.
   - Reassess.

3. All treatments begin with fascial techniques, to enable easier access to deeper tissues, to help reduce or eliminate superficial trigger points, and to begin accessing the global tissues being influenced by the areas you are working on. Working this way reduces the time taken to start making an impact.
   - These techniques are done with nothing but your clean, dry hands.
   - If patients have used body lotion, you will have to remove this before you start; I often use Zoff.

4. You will see that the techniques within this book are a combination of:
   - Myofascial release (MFR), which has lots of different names
   - Instrument-assisted soft-tissue mobilization (IASTM)
   - Trigger-point acupressure (waiting for the trigger-point pain to drop from VAS[2] 6/10 to 2/10)
   - Soft-tissue release (STR)—pin and stretch locks:
     - Transverse
     - Proximal
     - Distal
   - Active tissue release—pin and facilitate movement

   - Muscle energy techniques (MET)
     - Similar to proprioceptive neuromuscular facilitation (PNF) stretching, but not to true PNF
   - Dry needling (only for the qualified)
   - Dynamic taping

5. Not all these techniques will be needed—you will only need to tap into additional techniques if your reassessment produces no change. I have included lots of different techniques for your ever-growing "toolbox".

6. Be confident that once you have made a change you do not need to continually return to the same area—overtreatment is a pet hate of mine and has left many an athlete poorly prepared for training and competition.

7. You do not have to cause pain—avoiding pain enables you to work deeply without having the tissues physically refuse entry (see Chapter 2: Fascia), with the athlete gripping the edge of the plinth in agony or squirming to get away!
   - When sinking into tissues, ask the athlete to tell you when his or her discomfort level has reached 6/10 (VAS).
   - Hold this position until the athlete tells you that the discomfort has "dropped" or has reached the equivalent of 2/10 (VAS).
   - Add the movement, if appropriate; again holding the position if the discomfort level during the movement rises to 6/10, then continue the movement when the discomfort has subsided.
   - This will target any superficial and sometimes deeper trigger points, prior to activating the stretch or facilitation.
   - Once this tissue has been addressed, move to a point close to the original point, and repeat until all tissues in the area (or around the joint) have been addressed.

8. I use IASTM following my "dry" fascial and soft-tissue techniques, particularly around joints and hard-to-reach places, but also when I am looking for a more global response.
   - I use the Kinnective™ instrument because I can use the same instrument to do lots of techniques, and it feels great in my hand.
   - I also use Kinesiotech emollient, because I've tried quite a few and find this the least messy, and it smells divine.

---

1. T, thyroid; H, heart; R, rheumatoid arthritis; E, epilepsy; A, asthma; D, diabetes; O, osteoarthritis; C, Cancer.

2. Visual analogue scale for pain.

9. I have added dry needling (DN) techniques for those that are qualified and suitably insured; there are more, but the ones in this book are the ones I use regularly. I tend to resort to DN:
   ■ When all the soft-tissue work is done and my reassessment calls for that intervention
   ■ When the area is too painful (owing to trigger points) for direct manual techniques
   ■ When the area is being particularly stubborn, to avoid overtreating and damaging the tissues

10. When dry needling, I switch between:
    ■ Piston-type work (searching for the offending trigger points)
    ■ Fascial winding (affecting the global network)
    ■ Quick in and out (similar to the Gunn method)
    ■ Electroacupuncture (facilitating relaxation to hypertonic structures)

11. I use muscle energy techniques following targeted soft-tissue work and DN as an adjunct to facilitate additional tissue extensibility and influence joint range of movement.

12. I use Dynamic Tape® because it is simply the best on the market for versatility and elastic recoil—the results are palpable and visible to both me and the athletes I treat.
    ■ You will need to have something to remove the emollient if you have included IASTM in your treatment session.

13. At the end of the book you will find mobilization, stretching, and strengthening advice, which can be put into a home exercise program (HEP) and given to your patients. This section is not exhaustive, as there are many books and YouTube clips out there that cover these in much more detail.
    ■ I use a program called Rehabmypatient on a regular basis as it enables me to e-mail photographic drawings and videos of the exercises I would like my patients to do to help facilitate the work that we are doing together.

Acknowledgments

Thank you Jon Hutchings for approaching me at the first ever TherapyExpo (2013) and asking me if I would be prepared to write this book, and thank you John Gibbons for standing there and encouraging me to agree.

Thank you to my husband Rick, who is always there for me, and who has the ability to "manage" a wife who is the epitome of an overachiever. Never once has he asked why I do the things I do. I am always, always, greeted with, "OK, so how do you want to go about it?" I am excited by life and new ideas, and he is always right there with me, making it happen. Thank you Rick, I love you more than words can say.

Definition of "Overachiever"

Someone who is ambitious, driven, and motivated to do (and be) the best, with a unique mindset that keeps the brain on overdrive and a work ethic that keeps him or her one step ahead. Having high expectations and focused intensity.

Overachievers have high aspirations and like to "dream big." There's always a lot on their plate—their to-do lists are full and they have an abundance of ideas for future books, businesses, projects, and improvements. They see every moment as a valuable opportunity to invest in a worthwhile endeavor.

Thank you to my three children—Scott, Adam, and Britt—who have always supported a mother who left regularly to travel the globe with one team or another. I've missed birthdays and special occasions but I have never had the guilt card played—they have supported me tirelessly. There were times that I wobbled and the guilt began to creep in, particularly when I was travelling a lot and Britt was only five or six; these times were always accompanied by hugs of encouragement and "we'll be fine, it's only a few weeks." Thank you for being amazing—I am so proud of you all.

Thank you to my parents Heather and Ray Stott for allowing me to be me and encouraging me to achieve my dreams. Thank you for enabling me to move to the Canary Islands when I was nineteen to meet the man of my dreams.

Thank you to my lovely big brother Steve Stott, who has always been a real big brother to me. Thank you for teaching me so many things, despite my temper tantrums when I got frustrated and didn't understand. Thank you for saving me when I got stuck in the Thistlegorm wreck on our driving trip. Thank you for snapping that amazing shot of our encounter with the thresher shark.

Thank you to Ryan Kendrick for writing the chapter on Dynamic Tape®.

Thank you to Donna Strachan, who helped me compile the appendix: Instrument-Assisted Soft-Tissue Mobilization.

Thank you to Sophie Cook, who agreed to be my model for the photographs and to Liz Vanegas de Quickenden for taking them.

Finally, I would like to thank the many people who have inspired or supported me over the years—too many to mention but some that cannot go un-named (in no particular order): Alison Rose (roomy), Rone Thompson (roomy), Pierre McCourt, Angela McNaughton, Neil Black, Dr. Bruce Hamilton, Dr. Paul Dykstra, Dr. Robin Chakraverty, Dr. Gerry Ramogida, Denise Plimmer, and Amanda Stott.

References

Greenhalgh T, Howick J, and Maskrey N (2014) Evidence-based medicine: a movement in crisis? *British Medical Journal* 348(4): 3725–3725

Huntley AL, Johnson R, Purdy S, Valderas JM, and Salisbury C (2012) Measures of mulitmorbidity and morbidity burden for use in primary care and community settings: a systematic review and guide. *Annals of Family Medicine* 10(2): 134–141

Sackett DL, Rosenberg WMC, Gray JAM, Haynes RB, and Richardson WS (1996) Evidence-based medicine: what it is and what it isn't. *British Medical Journal* 312: 71–72

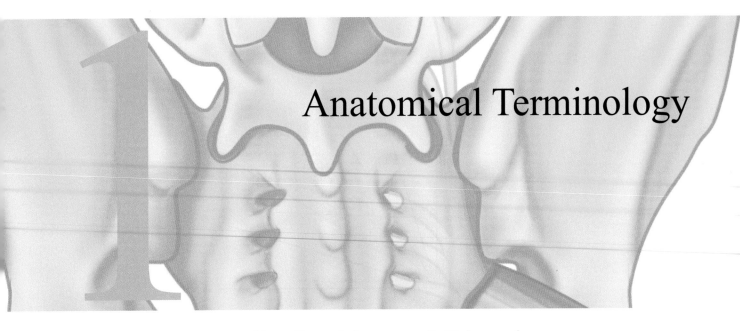

Anatomical Terminology

Terms to Describe Position and Direction

Anterior/ventral	Toward the front of the body
Posterior/dorsal	Toward the back of the body
Proximal/superior	Closer to the main mass of the body
Distal/inferior	Distant from the main mass of the body
Caudad	Toward the tail—similar to distal/inferior
Cephalad	Toward the head—similar to proximal/ superior
Deep	Beneath other structures
Superficial	Above other structures
Lateral	Away from the midline of the body
Medial	Toward the midline of the body
Palmar	Relating to the palm of the hand
Plantar	Relating to the sole of the foot
Prone	Lying face downward
Supine	Lying face upward
Flexion	Decreasing the angle between two body parts
Extension	Increasing the angle between two body parts
Adduction	Moving a body segment toward the midline
Abduction	Moving a body segment away from the midline
Horizontal abduction	Shoulders flexed at ninety degrees, moving in a transverse plane away from the front of the body
Horizontal adduction	Shoulders abducted to ninety degrees, moving in a transverse plane toward the midline of the body

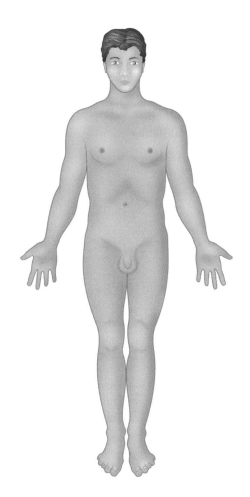

Figure 1.1: Universally accepted initial reference position to describe the relative positions of the body parts and their movements, known as the 'Anatomical Position'

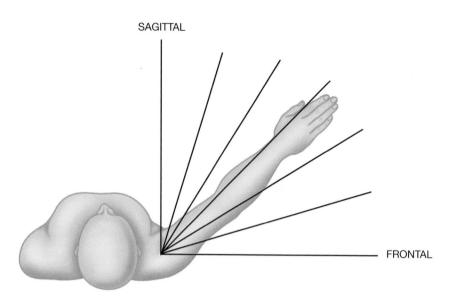

SAGITTAL

FRONTAL

Figure 1.2: Scapular plane

Scapular plane	Approximately thirty degrees from the midline between sagittal and frontal (see Figure 1.2)
Internal/medial rotation	Rotation toward the center of the body
External/lateral rotation	Rotation away from the center of the body
Circumduction	Combined flexion, extension, adduction, and abduction
Anterior translation	The movement of a body segment toward the front of the body in relation to the segments around it
Posterior translation	The movement of a body segment toward the back of the body in relation to the segments around it

Glossary

Agonists	Muscles that contract to move a body segment
Antagonists	Muscles that oppose a specific movement
Synergists	Muscles that perform, or help the agonist perform, the movement required, neutralizing excessive motion to ensure that the force generated is within the desired plane of movement
Ipsilateral	On the same side of the body
Contralateral	On the opposite side of the body
ASIS	Anterior superior iliac spine
AIIS	Anterior inferior iliac spine
PSIS	Posterior superior iliac spine
Rx	Treatment
Cx	Cervical spine
Tx	Thoracic spine
Lx	Lumbar spine
ROM	Range of movement
Overpressure	Passive end-of-range stretch without pain as a barrier
Crook lying	Lying with the knees flexed and feet on the plinth

VAS Pain Scale

The visual analogue scale (VAS) relates to the amount of pain that a patient feels, ranging across a continuum from no pain at all to an extreme amount of pain. Patients would circle the picture or mark on the line the point that they feel represents their perception of their current state (see Figure 1.3).

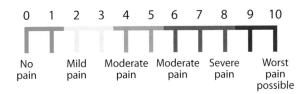

Figure 1.3: VAS pain scale

Planes of Motion

The term *plane* refers to a two-dimensional section through the body; it provides a view of the body or body part as though it has been cut through by an imaginary line (see Figure 1.4).

- The sagittal planes cut vertically through the body from anterior to posterior, dividing it into right and left halves.
- The frontal (coronal) planes pass vertically through the body, dividing it into anterior and posterior sections, and lie at right angles to the sagittal plane.
- The transverse planes are horizontal cross sections, dividing the body into upper (superior) and lower (inferior) sections, and lie at right angles to the other two planes.

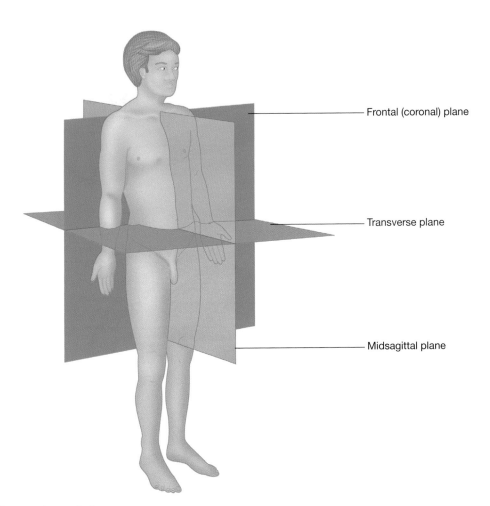

Figure 1.4: The most frequently used planes

Skeletal Muscle Structure and Function

Skeletal (somatic or voluntary) muscles make up approximately 40% of the total human body mass and consist of nonbranching striated muscle fibers, surrounded and held together by loose areolar tissue. The degree by which a muscle can shorten when it contracts is dependent on the arrangement of fibers within the muscle; although all movement is brought about by muscle shortening irrespective of muscle-fiber arrangement. The primary function of skeletal muscles is to produce movement, through their ability to contract, shorten, and consequently pull across joints to change the relative positions of the bones involved. Muscle tendons blend into the periosteum of a bone via fascial extensions (attachments).

Overview of Skeletal Muscle Structure

The functional unit of skeletal muscle is the muscle fiber (see Figure 1.5a). A muscle consists of many individual fibers, which are elongated cylindrical cells with multiple nuclei, ranging from ten to a hundred micrometers in width, and a few millimeters to over thirty centimeters (twelve inches) in length. The cytoplasm of the fiber is called the *sarcoplasm*, which is encapsulated inside a cell membrane called the *sarcolemma*. A delicate membrane known as the *endomysium* surrounds each individual fiber.

Muscle fibers are grouped together in bundles (see Figure 1.5b), or *fasciculi* (fascicles), covered by the *perimysium*. The bundles of muscle fibers are themselves grouped together, and the whole muscle is encased in a fascial sheath called the *epimysium*. These muscle membranes lie throughout the entire length of the muscle, from one attachment to the other. The whole structure is sometimes referred to as the *musculotendinous unit*.

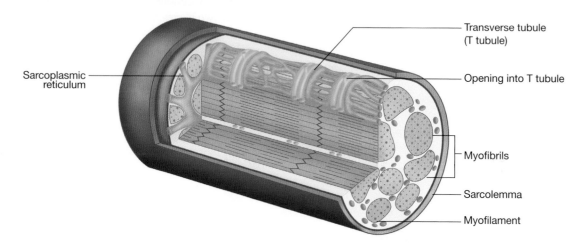

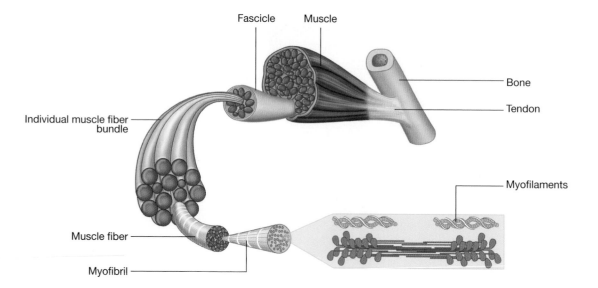

Figure 1.5: (a) Each skeletal muscle fiber is a single cylindrical muscle cell, (b) cross section of muscle tissue

Myofibrils

Through an electron microscope, one can distinguish the contractile elements of a muscle fiber, known as *myofibrils*, running the entire length of the fiber. Myofibrils are composed of long proteins including actin, myosin, titin, and other proteins that hold them together. These proteins are organized into thick and thin filaments called myofilaments, which repeat along the length of the myofibril in sections called sarcomeres. Muscles contract by sliding the thick (*myosin*) and thin (*actin*) filaments along each other. Myofibrils reveal alternate light and dark banding caused by the overlapping of the two different kinds of myofilaments, producing the characteristic cross-striation of the muscle fiber. The light bands are referred to as isotropic (I) bands and consist of thin actin myofilaments. The dark ones are called anisotropic (A) bands, consisting of thicker myosin myofilaments. A third connecting filament is made of the sticky protein *titin*, which is the third-most abundant protein in human tissue.

The myosin filaments have paddle-like extensions that emanate from the filaments, rather like the oars of a boat. These extensions latch onto the actin filaments, forming what are described as "cross-bridges" between the two types of filament. The cross-bridges, using the energy of adenosine triphosphate (ATP), pull the actin strands closer together[1]. Thus, the light and dark sets of filaments increasingly overlap, like an interlocking of the fingers, resulting in muscle contraction. One set of actin–myosin filaments is called a *sarcomere*.

---

1. The generally accepted hypothesis to explain muscle function is partly described by Hanson and Huxley's sliding filament theory (Huxley and Hanson, 1954). Muscle fibers receive a nerve impulse that causes the release of calcium ions stored in the muscle. In the presence of the muscle's fuel, ATP, the calcium ions bind with the actin and myosin filaments to form an electrostatic (magnetic) bond. This bond causes the fibers to shorten, resulting in their contraction or increase in tonus. When the nerve impulse ceases, the muscle fibers relax. Because of their elastic elements, the filaments recoil to their noncontracted lengths, i.e. their resting level of tonus.

Pennation/Fiber Orientation

Muscles come in a variety of shapes according to the arrangement of their fascicles. The reason for this variation is to provide optimum mechanical efficiency for a muscle in relation to its position and action. The most common arrangements of fascicles yield muscle shapes that can be described as parallel, pennate, convergent, and circular, with each of these shapes having further subcategories. The different shapes are illustrated in Figure 1.6.

Parallel

In this arrangement the fascicles run parallel to the long axis of the muscle. If the fascicles extend throughout the length of the muscle, it is known as a strap muscle—for example, the *sartorius*. If the muscle also has an expanded belly and tendons at both ends, it is called a fusiform muscle—for example, the *biceps brachii*. A variation of this type of muscle has a fleshy belly at either end, with a tendon in the middle; such muscles are referred to as digastric.

Pennate

Pennate muscles are so named because their short fasciculi are attached obliquely to the tendon, like the structure of a feather (Latin *penna* = "feather"). If the tendon develops on one side of the muscle, it is referred to as unipennate—for example, the *flexor digitorum longus* in the leg. If the tendon is in the middle and the fibers are attached obliquely from both sides, it is known as bipennate, a good example of which is the *rectus femoris*. If there are numerous tendinous intrusions into the muscle, with fibers attaching obliquely from several directions (thus resembling many feathers side by side), the muscle is referred to as multipennate; the best example is the middle part of the *deltoid* muscle.

Convergent

Muscles that have a broad origin with fascicles converging toward a single tendon, giving the muscle a triangular shape, are called convergent muscles. The best example is the *pectoralis major*.

Circular

When the fascicles of a muscle are arranged in concentric rings, the muscle is referred to as circular. All the sphincter skeletal muscles in the body are of this type; they surround openings, which they close by contracting. An example is the *orbicularis oculi*.

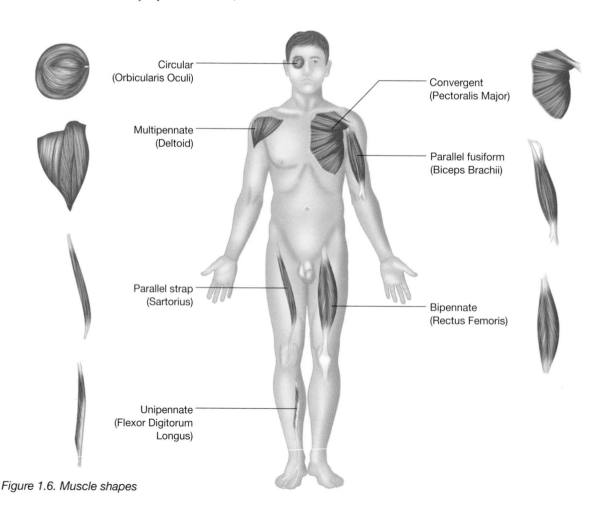

Figure 1.6. Muscle shapes

Nerve Tissue

Nervous tissue is composed of neurons. Neurons transmit nerve impulses. A neuron is made up of a cell body, an axon, and a dendrite. The axon resembles a long, thin wire that arises from the cell body. The dendrites are short protruding fibers that convey impulses toward the cell body.

The axon can have an outer covering called the myelin sheath. The diameter of this fatty covering is constricted at intervals along its length. These interruptions in the myelin are called nodes of Ranvier. Axons that have this outer covering are known as myelinated fibers, while those without it are called unmyelinated. Such fibers are found mostly in the autonomic nervous system. All axons have an outer covering called the neurolemma but this is only found on nerves outside the spinal cord.

The nervous system is sending signals to all the body's cells twenty-four hours a day. Neurons that connect the spinal cord (which typically ends between your first and second lumbar vertebrae) to the toes can be half a meter or longer. Nerves can be as thick as your little finger or as thin as a fine thread; in fact they can be microscopic.

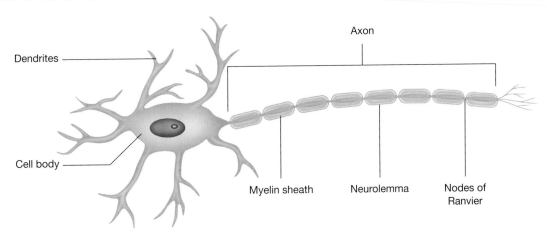

Figure 1.7: Nervous tissue and nerve cells

The Sciatic Nerve

The sciatic nerve is the longest and widest nerve in the human body. It originates in the lower back, from spinal nerves L4 through S3, and passes deeply to the piriformis muscle down to the lower limb. The sciatic nerve innervates biceps femoris, semimembranosus, and semitendinosus. True sciatic insults include changes in sensation, numbness, weakness, and even the sensation of water running down the limb. Depending on the source and level of irritation, the pain can be mild to severe. Sciatic nerve irritation usually occurs at the L5 or S1 level of the spine and only on one side. Pain can travel all the way to the foot and can retard normal motion, but with normal healing, the referred pain should dissipate and become more central. Unresolved chronic pain, especially of unknown origin, should be brought to the attention of the doctor or primary healthcare team.

Midway between the pelvis and the popliteal fossa, the sciatic nerve divides into the tibial nerve and the common fibular (peroneal) nerve.

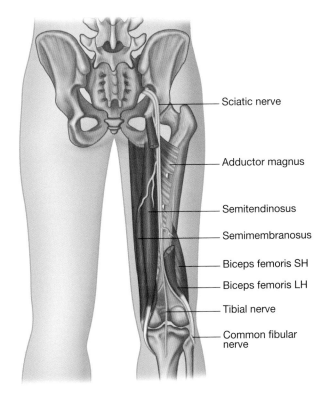

Figure 1.8: The sciatic nerve

Fascia

See Chapter 2: Fascia, for more information.

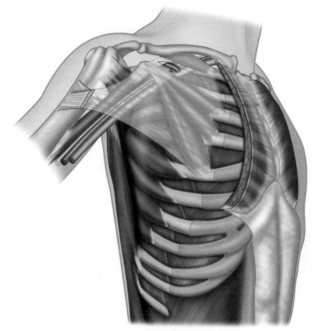

Figure 1.9: The fascial sheath

Posture

Posture is the body's way of maintaining balance and control with tiny active muscle contractions that are controlled by numerous mechanisms (elastic recoil in muscles, core muscles, higher control from the nervous system) and is fundamental to efficient movement.

When the body is balanced these small adjustments go unnoticed, taking minimal effort. When standing, sitting, or squatting, the body fluctuates to support itself against gravity, allowing the whole tensegrity structure to move and interact effectively in order to maintain balance.

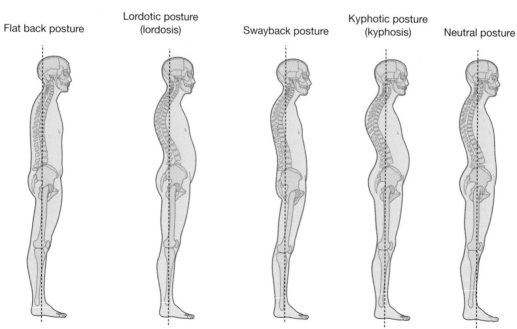

Flat back posture   Lordotic posture (lordosis)   Swayback posture   Kyphotic posture (kyphosis)   Neutral posture

Figure 1.10: Posture

Gait

Gait is a form of bipedal locomotion combining an alternating action between the lower extremities and a series of rhythmic alternating movements of the arms and trunk to create forward propulsion. One leg remains on the ground in order to restrain, support, and facilitate propulsion, whilst the other produces a swing phase (to create a step forward).

1. *Stance phase* (foot is on the ground, contributes to 60% of the gait cycle)
- Heel strike to foot flat
- Foot flat through midstance
- Midstance through to heel off
- Heel off to toe off

2. *Swing phase* (foot has no contact with the ground, contributes to 40% of the gait cycle)
- Acceleration to midswing
- Midswing to deceleration

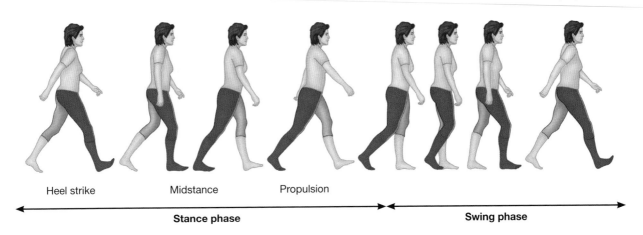

Heel strike   Midstance   Propulsion

Stance phase   Swing phase

Figure 1.11: Stance and swing phases of the gait cycle

Trendelenberg Gait

Trendelenberg gait is caused by weakness of the hip abductors (gluteus medius and minimus), and subsequent loss of their stabilizing effect. During the stance phase of gait, this weakness becomes apparent (in the coronal plane) when the pelvis on the contralateral side tilts downward (loss of pelvic stability) or the trunk compensates by shifting to the weaker side, attempting to maintain a level pelvis throughout the gait cycle (e.g. when standing on the left leg, the right hip drops = positive Trendelenberg).

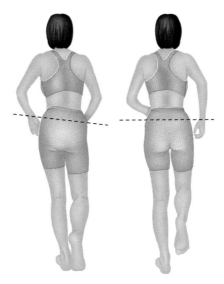

Figure 1.12: Trendelenberg gait

Nutation and Counternutation

It is well documented that there is very limited movement at the SIJ. The two main movements occur when the sacrum moves relative to the iliac bones in the sagittal plane. *Nutation* describes when the sacrum is rotated forward relative to the iliac bones (close packed position), and occurs in preparation for joint loading (see Figure 1.13a). *Counternutation* describes when the sacrum is rotated backwards relative to the iliac bones (see Figure 1.13b).

Pelvic Tilts

Anterior pelvic tilt is when the anterior superior iliac spine (ASIS) of the pelvis is positioned lower than in the anatomical position, and the posterior superior iliac spine (PSIS) is positioned higher (commonly caused by short hip flexors and lengthened hip extensors, increasing lumbar lordosis [anterior curvature of the spine]) (see Figure 1.14a).

Posterior pelvic tilt is when the ASIS of the pelvis is positioned higher than in the anatomical position and the PSIS is positioned lower (commonly caused by shortened hip extensors, particularly the gluteus maximus, and lengthened hip flexors, decreasing lumbar lordosis and producing a flat back) (see Figure 1.14b).

Lateral pelvic tilt is when one side of the pelvis is elevated above the other (common when a scoliosis [lateral deviation of the spine] is present or a leg-length discrepancy).

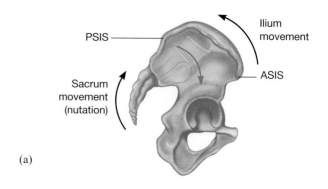

(a)

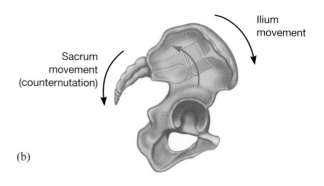

(b)

Figure 1.13: (a) Posterior pelvic rotation and sacral nutation; (b) anterior pelvic rotation and sacral counternutation

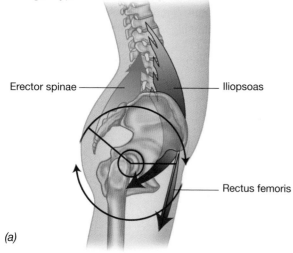

(a)

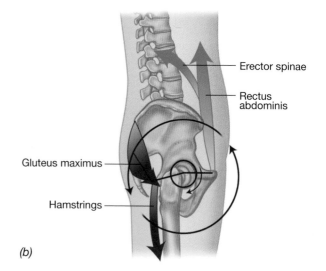

(b)

Figure 1.14: Pelvic tilt. (a) Direction of anterior tilt; (b) direction of posterior tilt

Reference

Huxley H and Hanson J (1954). Changes in the cross-striations of muscle during contraction and stretch and their structural interpretation. *Nature* 173(4412): 973–976

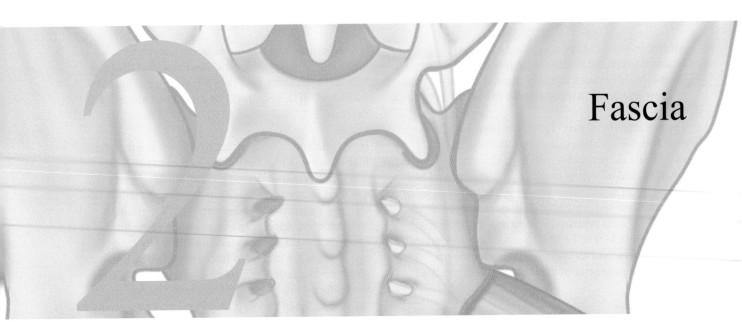

The information provided in this chapter may be a bit dry, but I feel it is important to try to understand why the techniques we use have the effects that they have.

Fascia has been defined as:

> [the] soft tissue component of the connective tissue system that permeates the human body ... effectively a network recognised as part of a body-wide tensional force transmission system.
> (Schleip et al., 2012)

> ... seamless integration seen in a living body. When one part moves, the body as a whole responds. Functionally, the only tissue that can mediate such responsiveness is the connective tissue.
> (Schultz and Feitis, 1996)

It is rare that muscles transmit their full force directly through tendons into the bones of the skeleton; in fact, they distribute a large portion of their contractile forces into fascial sheets (Findley, 2011). Muscles like the gluteus maximus have eighty-five percent of their fibers investing into the fascia lata (as opposed to the muscular insertion). Muscles also transmit forces laterally to neighboring muscles; in some cases, almost fifty percent of the muscle-generated force goes laterally rather than to the tendon (Maas and Sandercock, 2010; Findley, 2011). These forces go to the synergistic partners, as well as across the limb to antagonistic muscles. Thereby they not only stiffen the respective joint, but may even affect regions several joints away (Findley, 2011).

Components of Fascia

In general terms, fascia comes in two forms: dense deep connective tissue, offering high collagen, tensile strength, and stiffness, and areolar connective tissue.

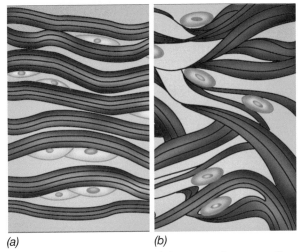

(a)   (b)

Figure 2.1: (a) The structure of dense regular connective tissue; (b) the structure of dense irregular connective tissue

Dense deep connective tissue has two types: dense regular connective tissue (see Figure 2.1a), where fibers travel in parallel arrangement along the lines of predominant force acting upon the tissue (tendons, ligaments, aponeuroses, intermuscular septa), and dense irregular connective tissue (see Figure 2.1b), which is meshlike, allowing resistance to stress in many different directions, enabling the tissue to resist unpredictable stress.

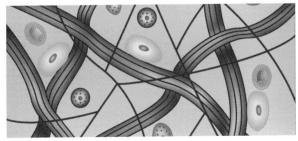

Figure 2.2: Loose connective tissue, e.g. areolar tissue

Areolar or loose connective tissue (with sparsely arranged fibers and strands, see figure 2.2) provides a flexible layer between layers of dense connective tissue to allow structures to move relative to one another.

The extracellular matrix (ECM) has been described as a dynamic complex that constantly modifies its viscoelastic properties; adapts to changes in physiological as well as mechanical demands; and is composed of a gelatinous ground substance made up of glycoproteins and proteoglycans, which is interwoven by stiffer fibrous proteins (Schleip and Baker, 2015) (see Figure 2.3). The ECM also serves as a mechanical buffer system, and its hydration can influence the mechanical properties of the ECM (Schleip and Baker, 2015).

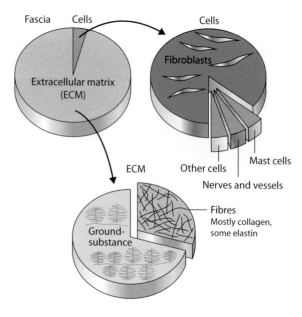

Figure 2.3: Components of fascia. The basic constituents are cells (mostly fibroblasts) and extracellular matrix, the latter of which consists of fibers plus the watery ground substance.
(Illustration courtesy of fascialnet.com)

It is widely accepted that the proteoglycans (extracellular proteins bound by polysaccharides called glycosaminoglycans (GAGs)) present in the ECM (ground substance) are there to facilitate mechanical strength and resistance to compression. These GAGs are negatively charged, which gives them hydrophilic (attracting water) properties. Ensuring correct water regulation and electrolyte balance of tissues is important to us as practitioners. The moving and sliding function of fascia has been described as being based on two features: its anatomical arrangement of parallel collagen and elastic fibers, and the presence of hyarulonic acid (HA) (Stecco et al., 2011). The biosynthesis and secretion of HA is performed by *fasciacytes*, according to Stecco et al. (2011). Polymerization, forming large

HA molecules, and depolymerization, breaking HA down into smaller molecules, allow fascia to fluctuate between a gel and a fluidlike (sol) state when heated (Schleip, 2003), as in direct treatment techniques or exercise.

Having an understanding that hydration, and therefore lubrication (vital for the gliding of tissues), prevents collagen fibers from forming cross-links (adhesions) and therefore reduces loss of movement and subsequent injury is imperative. Fundamentally, if the ground substance has inadequate water content at the time of injury or trauma, the body cannot efficiently absorb and disperse the impact of forces acting on it. It has also been suggested by Schleip and Baker (2015) that the profound effects reported following therapeutic skin taping (used in sports medicine) may be partially explained by its amplification of respective skin movements in normal joint functioning.

Just as movement and loading influence fascial tissue, so does immobilization. Immobility reduces the elasticity and gliding ability of the tissues (fiber arrangement becomes disorganized and multidirectional cross-linkages form), which in turn leads to tissue adhesions (Järvinen et al., 2002) (see Figure 2.4). Similarly, if functional or structural disturbances are present, the fascial continuity is disrupted, leading to altered tension in the myofascial network.

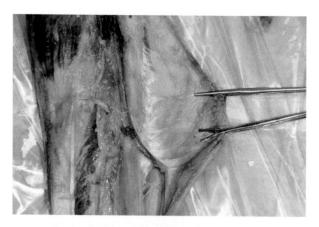

Figure 2.4: Immobility reduces the elasticity and gliding ability of the tissues, which leads to tissue adhesions (Image courtesy of John Sharkey, 2008)

It is essential to realize that approximately two-thirds of the volume of fascial tissues is made up of water. Loose connective tissue harbors the vast majority of the fifteen liters (nearly thirty-two pints) of interstitial fluid, and therefore regulates nutrient transport to metabolically active cells (Reed and Rubin, 2010). During application of mechanical load—whether in a stretching manner or via local compression—a significant amount of water is pushed out of the more stressed zones, similar to squeezing a sponge (Schleip et al., 2012). With the release that follows, this area is again filled with new fluid, which comes from surrounding tissue as well as the local vascular network. The spongelike connective tissue can lack adequate hydration at neglected places.

Application of external loading to fascial tissues can result in a refreshed hydration of such places in the body (Chaitow, 2009). In healthy fascia, a large percentage of the extracellular water is in a state of bound water, as opposed to bulk water (Pollack, 2013), where its behaviour can be characterized as that of a liquid crystal. Much pathology —such as inflammatory conditions, edema, or the increased accumulation of free radicals and other waste products—tends to go along with a shift towards a higher percentage of bulk water within the ground substance. When local connective tissue gets squeezed like a sponge (perhaps by interventions such as stretching or use of a foam roller) and subsequently rehydrated, some of the previous bulk water zones may then be replaced by bound water molecules, which could lead to a more healthy water constitution within the ground substance (Schleip et al., 2012; Pollack, 2013).

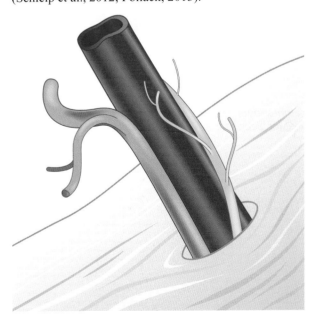

Figure 2.5: The superficial fascia will be perforated by structures such as arteries, veins, and nerves. (Illustration reproduced from Massage Fusion (Fairweather and Mari, 2015) with permission by Handspring Publishing))

The ability of fascia and associated structures to adapt to changes in shear force minimizes damage and allows varying degrees of forces to be transmitted smoothly and efficiently (Schleip et al., 2006). Fascia also creates compartments, dissipates stress concentration at the *entheses* (sites where the fascial surroundings of tendons or ligaments insert into the periosteum surrounding bones), and coordinates muscular activity and *proprioception* (the unconscious perception of movement and spatial orientation arising from stimuli within the body itself) (van der Wal, 2009).

It has been demonstrated that both free and encapsulated nerve endings are embedded within the deep fascia and that the fascia is richly innervated (van der Wal, 2009; Bhattacharya et al., 2010). We know that each muscle is enveloped by epimysium, which either consists of two parallel sets of wavy collagen embedded in a proteocollagen matrix in a crossed-ply arrangement (in some long, straplike muscles), or is arranged parallel to the long axis of the muscle, forming a dense surface layer that functions as a surface tendon (in pennate muscles) (Purslow, 2010). We also know that the perimysium (dividing muscles into fascicles or bundles) merges seamlessly into the epimysium and they are connected mechanically. The myotendinous junctions (MTJs) are formed by the interdigitation of the ends of these fascial structures. So, it stands to reason that the superficial fascia will be perforated by structures such as arteries, veins, and nerves (see figure 2.5) (Bhattacharya et al., 2010).

As therapists we can therefore understand that any compression or restriction within the fascial network can contribute to hypertonicity, pain, and weakness. We need to understand how this system works so that when we put our hands on people we know what we are trying to achieve in attempting to return a body from dysfunction to function.

Fascial tissues slowly and consistently react to everyday loading, as well as to specific load training, with the help of the fibroblasts (Kjaer et al., 2009). With challenges to the mechanical integrity of the ECM, particularly with repeated and regular challenges—to tissue strength, shearing ability, and extensibility— fibroblasts are stimulated to restructure and rearrange the fascial web (mechanotransduction). For manual therapists, it is important to understand the enormity and potential impact on their practice of the following statement: There is proven structural change occurring as a result of the conversion from mechanical loading to cellular response, with the application of manual compression load (soft-tissue techniques/foam roller) or through movement or stretch (Khan and Scott, 2009; Chaitow, 2013).

It is widely accepted that following contraction, muscles transmit up to forty percent of their force via fascial investment into the muscles positioned next to them (including force transmission to antagonistic muscles), and not into their tendons as originally thought (Huijing, 2007; Klinger and Schleip, 2015). Examples of this force transmission can be seen when looking at the relationships between the latissimus dorsi, the lumbodorsal fascia, and the contralateral gluteus maximus (Figure 2.6a) (Barker et al., 2004); the gluteus maximus, fascia lata, and lower leg muscles (Figure 2.6b) (Stecco et al., 2013); or the biceps femoris, sacrotuberous ligament, and erector spinae (Figure 2.6c) (Vleeming et al., 1995).

Despite clear evidence suggesting that the connective tissue in our bodies is able to withstand substantial load, it is apparent that in many clinical scenarios the connective tissue is subjected to mechanical loads that are far too low (Schleip and Baker, 2015). It is also clear that mechanical loading provides one of the strongest stimuli, if not the strongest, toward an adaptation of matrix tissue that becomes stronger and, in an injury recovery situation, heals faster and better than if no loading were present (Schleip and Baker, 2015).

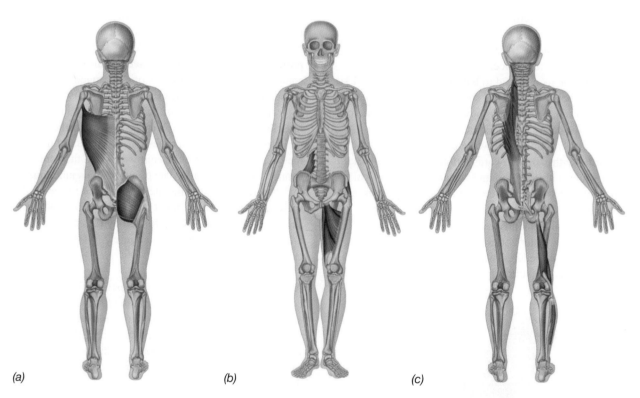

(a) (b) (c)

Figure 2.6: Examples of force transmission. (a) Latissimus dorsi, lumbodorsal fascia, and contralateral gluteus maximus; (b) gluteus maximus, fascia lata, and lower leg muscles; (c) biceps femoris, sacrotuberous ligament, and erector spinae

Tensegrity

Ingber (1993) stated that:

Only tensegrity can explain how every time that you move your arm, your skin stretches, your ECM extends, your cells distort, and the interconnected molecules that constitute the internal framework of the cell feel the pull—all without any breakage or discontinuity.

He went on to say:

An increase in tension of one of the members results in increased tension in members throughout the structure, even ones on the opposite side.

What Ingber is identifying here is the mechanical distribution of strain throughout the body. Therefore, any disruption to that network (damage to the soft tissues, no matter its location on the body, including overuse and postural adaptation) will be transmitted throughout the entire body (see Figure 2.7).

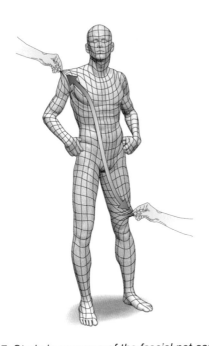

Figure 2.7: Strain in one area of the fascial net can be transmitted elsewhere in the body.
(Illustration reproduced from Massage Fusion (Fairweather and Mari, 2015) with permission by Handspring Publishing)

Evidence to Support the Principles of Tensegrity

Kassolik et al. (2009) recently conducted a study to investigate the transmission of tension through the body, based on the principle of tensegrity. They repeated a short massage on the brachioradialis and peroneal muscles of thirty-three participants, three times. Despite not being connected directly to the muscles being massaged, the deltoid and the tensor fasciae latae muscles responded to the massage (the former to massage of the brachioradialis, the latter to that of the peroneals), thereby confirming the principle of tensegrity.

Anatomy Trains

Myers (1997, 2001, 2009) found that the whole fascial network was divided into functional lines or kinetic chains of myofascia. He classified each line according to its movement functions, and found that localized injuries within a certain line transmitted tension along that line (leading to the subsequent dysfunction of that entire line and, indeed, many of the other lines). Myers recommended balancing the lines through myofascial manual therapy (impacting on the body as a whole functional unit and minimizing the previous effects of injuries), thereby reducing the risk of future injuries and improving the overall movement function of the body.

Preparing for sports performance includes specific repetitive training. Technical training, owing to its repetitive nature, will produce a loading response in the fascial tissue (thickening); if adaptation to that load does not occur and is not addressed, movement will be affected. When efficiency is affected, imbalances in strength and endurance of the tissues follow (Chaitow, 2007; De Witt and Venter, 2009). De Witt and Venter (2009) assessed muscle lengths of elite athletes and found that stabilizing muscles became "locked long" with repetitive use, while the more powerful muscles become "locked short."

Bunkie Test

De Witt and Venter (2009) proposed the Bunkie test as an outcome measure to identify fascial restrictions in five functional lines, after they noticed that repetitive movements could cause the fascia to respond by shortening and thickening or lengthening in opposing tissues (leading to dysfunction and injury). Developed over twelve years of working with elite athletes, this isometric test was used to identify where fascial restrictions were apparent and in which kinetic chains and along which fascial lines (Myers, 2009). If the fascia is fully functional in a specific line, it should allow all the muscles in that line to activate and support the body in the test position (forty seconds) for that line. If not, and if burning, stinging, or any discomfort limits the time in the specific position, a restricted or "locked long" area is indicated. Recommendations are that the test be repeated regularly after intervention until all positions can be held for forty seconds.

Recent interest, particularly in athletic populations, in the Bunkie test amongst physical therapists (Brumitt, 2009) and strength and conditioning coaches (Ronai, 2015) should also be noted, despite the test not having been assessed (as yet) for reliability and validity.

The Bunkie Test—Practical Application

- *Five positions/functional lines*
- Repeated on left and right sides of the body
- Equipment needed:
    - Bench, ten to twelve inches (25–30 cm) high
    - Nonslip mat
    - Stopwatch
- Each position held for forty seconds (athletes)
- Athletes who have neutral balanced fascia will be able to hold all five of these positions for forty seconds on both legs without feeling any strain
- Test stopped if cramping, burning, or pain is felt (this is not a strength test)
- Time recorded
- Do not do this test if you have had joint surgery in the past three months
- Should show improvement within first three sessions—need an experienced fascial therapist
- All Rx (treatment) techniques can be tested for effectiveness with the Bunkie test
- Determines which areas are locked long and are therefore weaker
- Immediate pain = locked long fascia/muscles inhibited
- Burning/cramping/pain/strain = diminished mobility of fascia on that line
    - Rx—average four times, twice per week

Example:
> *Monday—Rx prior to training and Rx following training*
> *Thursday—same*

- Weak lines/cannot hold position owing to weakness rather than pain or discomfort?
    - Activate prior to training
    - Hold weak lines two times, two seconds— build up to six times, six seconds, etc.

Posterior Power Line

- Maintain shoulders and hips in line
- Elbows placed perpendicularly to shoulders
- No rotation allowed
- Hands must not be under the hips offering support
- Ankle held in plantigrade
- Hold for forty seconds/record score on the initiation of any discomfort.

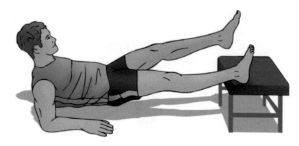

Figure 2.8: The posterior power line

Posterior Stabilizing Line

- Maintain shoulders and hips in line
- Elbows placed perpendicularly to shoulders
- Keep knees in ninety degrees of flexion
- No rotation allowed
- Hands must not be under the hips offering support
- Ankle held in plantigrade
- Hold for forty seconds/record score on the initiation of any discomfort.

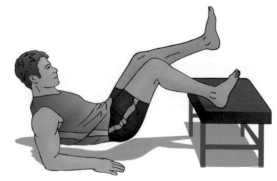

Figure 2.9: The posterior stabilizing line

Anterior Power Line

- Maintain shoulders and hips in line
- Elbows placed perpendicularly to shoulders
- Forearms must face forward and be parallel to one another
- Hands must not be under the hips offering any support
- Hold for forty seconds (athletes).

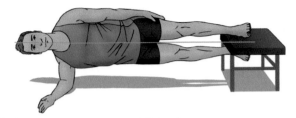

Figure 2.12: The medial stabilizing line

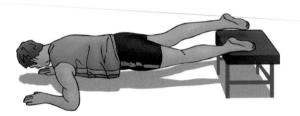

Figure 2.10: The anterior power line

Lateral Power Line

- Maintain shoulders and hips in line
- Elbow placed perpendicularly to shoulder
- Contralateral arm placed along contralateral side, hand resting on hip
- No rotation or tilting allowed
- Legs must be fully extended
- Ankles held in plantigrade
- Hold for forty seconds/record score on the initiation of any discomfort.

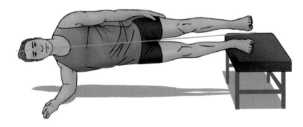

Figure 2.11: The lateral power line

Medial Stabilizing Line

- Maintain shoulders and hips in line
- Elbow placed perpendicularly to shoulder
- Contralateral arm placed along contralateral side, hand resting on hip
- No rotation or tilting allowed
- Legs must be fully extended
- Lower foot should be held against the bench
- Ankles held in plantigrade
- Hold for forty seconds/record score on the initiation of any discomfort.

Optimal muscle function is required for complex and repetitive movement patterns in sport. Therefore, it is important for coaches and therapists to be able to test for all the factors impacting and influencing that muscle function, including fascial restrictions. The Bunkie test was designed to test fascial restrictions along kinetic chains and could be the ideal tool for coaches and therapists to confirm that an athlete can return to his or her sport. Whilst I have focused on the sporting population, I also use this test regularly when treating the general public.

The Pelvis

An examination of the fascial characteristics to local and stability challenges affecting lumbopelvic "stability" and pelvic-girdle or lower-back pain is beneficial and instructive in how the central nervous system interacts for optimum motor control (Schleip and Baker, 2015). The key role that the pelvis plays as the link between the trunk and lower limbs should be acknowledged (Cusi, 2010), along with the fact that pelvic-girdle or sacroiliac incompetence can have a correlation with lower-back pain, injury, incontinence, and breathing issues (Schleip and Baker, 2015).

Sacroiliac joint (SIJ) stabilization is enhanced by the specific extensive myofascial contributions to force closure and ligamentous tensioning; for example, the sacrotuberous ligament (van Wingerden et al., 2004). Force closure has been defined as:

> *the effect of changing joint reaction forces, generated by tension in ligaments, fasciae and muscles, and ground reaction forces in order to overcome the forces of gravity by the provision of strong compression.*
> *(Cusi, 2010)*

Beneficial force transmission exists in the extensive connections of the gluteus maximus, biceps femoris, latissimus dorsi, paraspinal muscles, transversus abdominis/internal oblique aponeurosis, and the thoracolumbar fascia (Carvalhais et al., 2013). The thoracolumbar fascia is critical to the integrity of the inferior lumbar spine and the SIJ (Willard et al., 2012). The SIJs are critical to smooth movement and are essential for effective load transfer between the spine and the limbs, the functional interactions and slings mentioned above (Cusi, 2010; Vleeming et al., 2012).

Treatment Considerations

Prior to any connective-tissue or fascial treatment intervention, I strongly recommend assessing your athlete's hydration status. As previously discussed, chronic stress by dehydration and immobility causes excessive bonding, leading to the formation of scars and adhesions and limiting the movement of these usually resilient tissues.

As clinicians you will be completing full subjective and objective assessments prior to any treatment intervention. We would not want to focus all of our attention on the area of complaint; we would be looking to implement a global treatment pain-reduction program. The objective assessment process should include observational and palpatory (at velocities consistent with thixotropic properties of the tissue) joint and muscle testing, as well as outcome measures such as the Bunkie test.

Skillful application of manual forces on the fascial system conditions and reverses collagen overproduction processes, thus improving tissue functionality and optimizing rehabilitation mechanisms of musculoskeletal injuries (Martinez Rodriguez and Galan del Rio, 2015).

However, when the athlete is experiencing a state of high local and general fascial pre-tension, which is frequently observed in a sporting context, it will prove necessary to include within prevention and treatment intervention techniques specifically addressed to increasing elasticity and deformation capacity of stiff fascial areas (Schleip and Baker, 2015). Classical rehabilitation programs comprise pain-free stretching practices and other techniques specifically directed at the restricted area, such as deep friction massage, the Graston technique, and shock-wave therapy (Hammer, 2008; Sussmich-Leitch et al., 2012). However, these measures might prove insufficient. In this context, it becomes apparent that there is a need to apply skillful manual forces over the restricted areas in order to restore and improve the fascial system's capacity to absorb and dissipate repetitive mechanical loads (Martinez Rodriguez and Galan del Rio, 2015).

Myofascial injuries become highly scarred (pathological cross-links of collagen) with a high risk of re-injury (Baoge et al., 2012). This scarred area has formed owing to the damaged tissue's adaptation to early multidirectional loading. It is commonplace in sports medicine to treat scar tissue with PRP (platelet-rich

plasma) in order to speed up the healing process (Creaney and Hamilton, 2008). However, connective tissue proliferation excess, associated with the release of different growth factors, might decisively impair the achievement of an adequate regeneration–fibrosis balance and retractile scar formation, thereby resulting in functional deficiencies (Martinez Rodriguez and Galan del Rio, 2015). Manual treatment is recommended in this context (high-tension matrix), which is grounded in the need to accomplish a restoration of the preinjury status of damaged tissue, avoiding excessive collagen proliferation (Martinez Rodriguez and Galan del Rio, 2015). Facilitation of the tissues moving from a high-tension state to a lower-tension one is what we are attempting to influence. It is recommended that different mechanical stimuli be manually performed in a controlled way (directed manual mechanotransduction), as this results in tensional normalization at the microscopic level (tensional reharmonization between the cytoskeleton and the ECM through receptor integrins) (Martinez Rodriguez and Galan del Rio, 2013).

This reharmonization should enable cell-function normalization and should provide medium-term remodeling of the ECM (Martinez Rodriguez and Galan del Rio, 2013). Tozzie (2012) contributes to this discussion by stating that manual therapy decreases cross-links between collagen fibers with the possibility of influencing structural changes in fibrotic tissues. Schleip (2003) credits the benefits of fascial techniques to neurophysiological effects (modulations at different levels of the nervous system) via stimulation of mechanoreceptors, which are responsive to manual pressure and deformation. This is an important finding, as this direct-treatment method may facilitate the gliding of tissues owing to increased hydration (vasomotor reaction).

From a global rehabilitative approach, fascial techniques allow the collagen's restructuring capacity to increase prior to the execution of strength and stretching exercises. This is aimed at encouraging the longitudinal arrangement of the collagen's and fibroblasts' tension axes; the application of eccentric loads on deformable matrices presenting a smaller number of pathological cross-links and better hydration within fascial interfaces. This makes more sense than performing loading therapy on rigid matrices with weak sliding capacity between fascial layers (Martinez Rodriguez and Galan del Rio, 2015).

Myofascial injuries and the subsequent loss of range of movement (ROM) are commonly rehabilitated using stretching techniques and joint mobilization. These techniques do not fully take into consideration that immobilization following injury and pain causes the connective tissues investing into the joint (ligaments, capsule, periosteum) to become disorganized, dehydrate, and lose their elastic capacity. In addition, the gliding (between fascial layers), translation, and rotational capacity (of articular surfaces) is reduced significantly. Utilizing soft-tissue techniques that influence the periarticular system (scar-tissue techniques, deep tissue massage, deep frictions, neuromuscular techniques) to induce rehydration of the ground substance (thixotropic reaction) and rupture pathological cross-links prior to any direct joint mobilization and subsequent progressive loading would therefore be beneficial.

Stiffness within periarticular myofascial tissues may alter muscle tone regulation, negatively influence protocols designed for muscle strengthening, and alter proprioceptive re-education (fascial tissue is a substrate of proprioception) and training for restoration of sports-based movements (Stecco et al., 2007; van der Wal, 2009; Martinez Rodriguez and Galan del Rio, 2015). Mechanoreceptors are highly sensitive to minute tension variations, which are reflected throughout the entire fascial network. If this highly sensitive deformation detector is disrupted by injury and subsequent disorganization and stiffness of the damaged tissues, its capacity to respond with adaptation to traction, torsion, or compression forces may also be threatened. Martinez Rodriguez and Galan del Rio (2015) emphasize the importance of manual structural techniques to normalize the stimulatory mechanism of the mechanoreceptors (enabling effective motor response) and encourage rearrangement and remodeling of fascial architecture, prior to and during strengthening, loading, and proprioceptive training sessions. These techniques are noninvasive and effective, even on fascial areas remote to the pain, with an ability to modify the ECM and restore gliding (Stecco and Day, 2010).

McGlone et al. (2014) have found an interesting correlation between humans and other primates in the so-called "tactile C-fibers" in the superficial fascia (interstitial neurons present where furry skin would have been, evolutionarily associated with grooming behavior). When stimulated, these intrafascial neurons do not signal any proprioceptive information (and the brain cannot apparently locate the regional origin of the stimulation); however, they trigger activation in the insular cortex, which is expressed as a sense of peaceful well-being and social belonging (McGlone et al., 2014). Once again, this supports the use of manual therapy techniques and therapeutic massage.

Stretching

Lederman (2013) states that to influence ROM adaptation, physical activity intensity and duration need to lead to overload (beyond the current level). Often these thresholds are well above the levels experienced during functional daily activities (Muijka and Padilla, 2001; Arampatizis et al., 2010). Katalinic et al. (2010) concluded that clinical stretching (including passive and active) did not stimulate ROM adaptation, owing to the fact that many clinical stretching approaches did not provide the necessary force or were performed too quickly. Lederman (2013) recommends moving toward more functional approaches that integrate ROM into normal daily tasks.

References

Arampatizis A, Peper A, Bierbaum S and Albracht K (2010) Plasticity of human Achilles tendon mechanical and morphological properties in response to cyclic strain. *Journal of Biomechanics* 43(6): 3073–3079

Baoge L, van den Steen E, Rimbaut S, Philips N, Witvrouw E, Almqvist K, Vandersraeten G and Vanden Bossche L (2012) Treatment of skeletal muscle injury: a review. ISRN *Orthopaedics* 2012: 1–7

Barker PJ, Briggs CA and Bogeski G (2004) Tensile transmission across the lumbar fasciae in unembalmed cadavers: effects of tension to various muscular attachments. *Spine* 29(2): 129–138

Bhattacharya V, Barooah P, Nag,T, Chaudhuri G and Bhattacharya S (2010) Detail microscopic analysis of deep fascia of lower limb and its surgical implication. *Indian Journal of Plastic Surgery* 43(2): 135

Brumitt J (2009) A new functional test promoted to measure core strength. *NCSA's Performance Training Journal* 8(3): 15–16

Carvalhais VOD, Ocarino JM, Araujo VL, Souza TR, Silva PL and Fonseca ST (2013) Myofascial force transmission between the latissimus dorsi and gluteus maximus muscles: an in vivo experiment. *Journal of Biomechanics* 46: 1003–1007

Chaitow L (2007) *Positional Release Techniques.* Edinburgh: Churchill Livingstone

Chaitow L (2013) Understanding mechanotransduction and biotensegrity from an adaptation perspective. *Journal of Bodywork and Movement Therapies* 17: 141–142

Creaney L and Hamilton B (2008) Growth factor delivery methods in the management of sports injuries: the state of play. *British Journal of Sports Medicine* 42(5): 314–320

Cusi MF (2010) Paradigm for assessment and treatment of SIJ mechanical dysfunction. *Journal of Bodywork and Movement Therapies* 14: 152–161

De Witt B and Venter R (2009) The "Bunkie" test: assessing functional strength to restore function through fascia manipulation. *Journal of Bodywork and Movement Therapies* 13: 81–88

Fairweather R and Mari M (2015) *Massage Fusion.* Edinburgh: Handspring

Findley TW (2011) Fascia research from a clinician/scientist's perspective. *International Journal of Therapeutic Massage and Bodywork* 4(4): 1–6

Hammer WI (2008) The effect of mechanical load on degenerated soft tissue. *Journal of Bodywork and Movement Therapies* 12(3): 245–256

Huijing PA (2007) Epimuscular myofascial force transmission between antagonistic and synergistic muscles can explain movement limitation in spastic paresis. *Journal of Electromyographical Kinesiology* 17(6): 708–724

Ingber DE (1993) Cellular tensegrity: defining new rules of biological design that govern the cytoskeleton. *Journal of Cellular Science* 104(3): 613–627

Järvinen TAH, Józsa L, Kannus P, Järvinen TLN and Järvinen M (2002) Organization and distribution of intramuscular connective tissue in normal and immobilized skeletal muscles. *Journal of Muscle Research and Cell Motility* 23: 245–254

Kassolik K, Jaskólska A, Kisiel-sajewicz K, Marusiak J, Kawczyn´ski A and Jaskólski A (2009) Tensegrity principle in massage demonstrated by electro- and mechanomyography. *Journal of Bodywork and Movement Therapies* 13: 164–170

Katalinic OM, Harvey LA, Herbert RD (2010) Stretch for the treatment and prevention of contractures. Cochrane Database Systematic Review 8(9): CD007455

Khan KM and Scott A (2009) Mechanotherapy: how physical therapists' prescription of exercise promotes tissue repair. *British Journal of Sports Medicine* 43: 247–252

Kjaer M, Langberg H, Heinemeier K, Bayer ML, Hanse M, Holm L, Doessing S, Kongsgaard M, Krogsgaard MR and Magnusson SP (2009) From mechanical loading to collagen synthesis, structural changes and function in human tendon. *Scandinavian Journal of Medical Sports Science* 19(4): 500–510

Klinger W and Schliep R (2015) Fascia as a body-wide tensional network: anatomy, biomechanics and physiology. In Schleip R and Baker *A Fascia in Sport and Movement.* Edinburgh: Handspring

Lederman E (2013) *Therapeutic Stretching: Towards a Functional Approach.* London: Elsevier

Maas H and Sandercock TG (2010) Force transmission between synergistic skeletal muscles through connective tissue linkages. *Journal of Biomedicine and Biotechnology* 2010: 1–9

Martinez Rodriguez R and Galan del Rio F (2013) Mechanistic basis of manual therapy in myofascial injuries: sonoelastographic evolution control. *Journal of Bodywork and Movement Therapies* 17(2): 221–234

Martinez Rodriguez R and Galan del Rio F (2015) Understanding mechano-adaptation of fascial tissues: application to sports medicine. In Schleip R and Baker *A Fascia in Sport and Movement.* Edinburgh: Handspring

McGlone F, Wessberg J and Olausson H (2014) Discriminative and affective touch: sensing and feeling. *Neuron* 82(4): 737–755

Muijka M and Padilla S (2001) Muscular characteristics of detraining in humans. *Medical Science in Sports and Exercise* 333: 1297–1303

Myers TW (1997) The "anatomy trains": part 2. *Journal of Bodywork and Movement Therapies* 1(3): 134–145

Myers TW (2001) *Anatomy Trains*. Edinburgh: Churchill Livingstone

Myers TW (2009) *Anatomy Trains: Myofascial Meridians for Manual and Movement Therapists*. Edinburgh: Churchill Livingstone

Pollack GH (2013) *The Fourth Phase of Water: Beyond Solid, Liquid and Vapor*. Seattle, Washington: Ebner and Sons

Purslow P (2010) Muscle fascia and force transmission. *Journal of Bodywork and Movement Therapies* 14: 411–417

Reed RK and Rubin K (2010) Transcapillary exchange: role and importance of the interstitial fluid pressure and the extracellular matrix. *Cardiovascular Research* 87(2): 211–217

Ronai S (2015) The Bunkie Test. *Strength and Conditioning Journal* 37(3): 89–92

Schleip R (2003) Fascial plasticity—a new neurobiological explanation: parts I and II. *Journal of Bodywork and Movement Therapies* 7(1): 11–19

Schleip R and Baker A (2015) *Fascia in Sport and Movement*. Edinburgh: Handspring

Schleip R, Duerselen L, Vleeming A, Naylor IL, Lehmann-Horn F, Zorn A, Jaeger H and Klingler W (2012) Strain hardening of fascia: static stretching of dense fibrous connective tissues can induce a temporary stiffness increase accompanied by enhanced matrix hydration. *Journal of Bodywork and Movement Therapies* 16(1): 94–100

Schleip R, Naylor IL, Ursu D, Melzer W, Zorn A, Wilke HJ, Lehmann-Horn F and Klingler W (2006) Passive muscle stiffness may be influenced by active contractility of intramuscular connective tissue. *Medical Hypotheses* 66(1): 66–71

Schultz R and Feitis R (1996) *The Endless Web*. Berkeley, California: North Atlantic Books

Stecco A, Gilliar W, Hill R, Fullerton B and Stecco C (2013) The anatomical and functional relation between gluteus maximus and fascia lata. *Journal of Bodywork and Movement Therapies* 17(4): 512–517

Stecco C, Cagey O, Belloni A, Pozzuoli A, Porzionato A, Macchi V, Aldergheri R, DeCaro R and Delmas V (2007) Anatomy of the deep fascia of the upper limb—second part: study of innervation. *Morphologie* 91(292): 38–43

Stecco C and Day JA (2010) The fascial manipulation technique and its biomechanical model: a guide to the human fascial system. *International Journal of Therapeutic Massage and Bodywork* 3(1): 38–40

Stecco C, Stern R, Porzionato A, Macchi V, Masiero S, Stecco A and De Caro R (2011) Hyaluronan within fascia in the etiology of myofascial pain. *Surgery of Radiological Anatomy* 33(10): 891–896

Sussmich-Leitch SP, Collins NJ, Bialocerkowski AE, Warden SJ and Crossley KM (2012) Physical therapies for Achilles tendinopathy: systematic review and meta-analysis. *Journal of Foot and Ankle Research* 5(15): 1146–1162

Tozzie P (2012) Selected fascial aspects of osteopathic practice. *Journal of Bodywork Movement Therapies* 16(4): 503–519

van der Wal J (2009) The architecture of the connective tissue in the musculoskeletal system: an often overlooked functional parameter as to proprioception in the locomotor apparatus. *International Journal of Therapeutic Massage and Bodywork* 2(4): 9–23

van Wingerden JP, Vleeming A, Buyruk HM and Raissadat K (2004) Stabilisation of the sacroiliac joint in vivo: verification of muscular contribution to force closure of the pelvis. *European Spine Journal* 13:199–205

Vleeming A, Pool-Goudzwaard AL, Stoeckart R, van Wingerden JP and Snijders CJ (1995) The posterior layer of the thoracolumbar fascia: its function in load transfer from spine to legs. *Spine* 20(7): 753–758

Vleeming A, Schuenke MD, Masi AT, Carreiro JE, Danneels L and Willard FH (2012) The sacroiliac joint: an overview of its anatomy, function and potential clinical implications. *Journal of Anatomy* 221(6): 537–567

Willard FH, Vleeming A, Schuenke MD, Danneels L and Schleip R (2012) The thoracolumbar fascia: anatomy, function and clinical considerations. *Journal of Anatomy* 22(6): 507–536

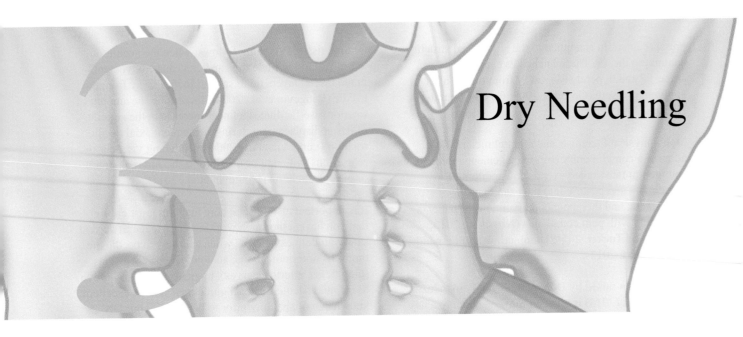

Dry Needling

I wanted to add a little something about dry needling (DN) because today many therapists practice DN as an adjunct to their manual techniques (when it falls within their scope of practice). Trigger-point dry needling (TPDN) is an invasive procedure in which an acupuncture needle (a fine filiform needle with small diameter) punctures the skin and is directed toward a myofascial trigger point (TP), allowing a unique interaction between the needle and the connective tissue (Langevin et al., 2001).

DN is a common treatment technique in orthopedic manual physical therapy (Dommerholt, 2011). Although various DN approaches exist, the more common and best-supported approach targets myofascial TPs from a pain-science perspective: trigger points are constant sources of peripheral nociceptive[1] input leading to peripheral and central sensitization. DN cannot only reverse some aspects of central sensitization, it reduces local and referred pain, improves range of motion and muscle-activation patterns, and alters the chemical environment of trigger points (Dommerholt, 2011).

Simons et al. (1999) defined the TP as:

A hyper-irritable spot in a taut band of a skeletal muscle that is painful on compression, stretch, overload or contraction of the tissue which usually responds with a referred pain that is perceived distant from the spot.

TPs constitute one of the most common musculoskeletal pain conditions (Hidalgo-Lozano et al., 2010; Bron et al., 2011), and are a regular source of nociceptive input (Ge and Arendt-Nielsen, 2011), influencing muscle-activation patterns, resulting in poor muscle coordination and balance (Lucas et al., 2010). Elimination of that peripheral input is necessary in order to restore lost coordination and balance.

One of the most distinguishing features of TPs is that they are located within taut bands (contracture within a few muscle fibers, independent of electrogenic activity) and do not involve the whole muscle (Simons and Mense, 1998; Chen et al., 2007; Rha et al., 2011). These taut bands are thought to be the product of local muscle overload, following excessive eccentric or concentric loading, where the muscle is unable to respond adequately to that load, potentially leading to a local energy crisis (Gerwin, 2008; Mense and Gerwin, 2010). Submaximal contractions in the neck and shoulders (upper trapezius muscles) of office workers are also found to produce TPs (Treaster et al., 2006; Hoyle et al., 2011).

The pH directly surrounding the TP is sufficiently low (well below five) to stimulate nociceptors (Gautam et al., 2010). The muscle, therefore, responds to stimuli such as light pressure and muscle movement, which leads to referred pain (Dommerholt and Fernandez-de-las-Penas, 2013).

Myofascial TPs are a common musculoskeletal complaint (Hidalgo-Lozano et al., 2010; Bron et al., 2011), which can occur with or without underlying pathology (Freeman et al., 2009). Active TPs refer pain, either locally or to another location elsewhere in the body along the nerve pathways, and a local twitch response is often detected (Rha et al., 2011). Latent TPs do not yet refer pain actively, but may do so when

---

1. The ability of a body to sense potential harm.

pressure or strain is applied to the myofascial structure containing the TP. These latent TPs cause allodynia[2] at the TP and hyperalgesia[3] away from the TP after applying pressure (Ge et al., 2008; Ge and Arendt-Nielsen, 2011).

Many physical therapists and other clinicians have adopted a contemporary pain-management approach and incorporate graded exercise, restoration of movement, and posture into the examination, assessment, and therapeutic interventions of patients presenting with pain complaints (Nijs et al., 2010; Hodges and Tucker, 2011; Dommerholt and Fernandez-de-las-Penas, 2013).

One question raised by Dommerholt and Fernandez-de-las-Penas (2013) is whether movement approaches by themselves are sufficient to address persistent pain states without eliminating peripheral nociceptive input. Mosely (2003, 2012) states that pain is produced by the brain when danger is perceived by the body, and that the brain requires an action to remove that pain. Therefore, the desired effect of DN to reduce pain cannot be considered without taking into consideration the biopsychosocial model (Gerwin and Dommerholt, 2006), particularly in persistent pain conditions (Melzack, 2001; Ge and Arendt-Nielsen, 2011) and abnormal movement patterns (Lucas et al., 2004, 2010).

Over recent years, a substantial amount of research surrounding the mechanisms by which acupuncture may decrease pain from a scientific perspective has been produced. This has revealed possible analgesic effects due to cortical responses in the somatosensory, limbic, basal ganglia, brain stem, and cerebellar regions, suggesting that the mechanisms by which acupuncture may alter pain are neuromodulatory (Huang et al., 2012; McGrath and White, 2015). Napadow et al. (2007) demonstrated that scanning while needling showed activation of the hypothalamus and deactivation in the amygdala (both involved in pain processing). When treating patients/athletes, how you explain what you are doing is imperative; language that blames local muscle pathology as being solely responsible for persistent pain should be avoided (Nijs et al., 2010; Puentedura and Louw, 2012).

During TPDN, the needle pierces the skin and passes through superficial and deep fascia (Langevin and Huijing, 2009; Findley, 2012). If the needle is rotated once it is inserted, collagen bundles are pulled and gathered from the periphery, causing this connective tissue to wrap around the needle's shaft (Langevin et al., 2002) (see Figure 3.1). A form of sustained localized

internal tissue stretching follows, when the needles are left in situ to facilitate this, and can cause movement in the fascial layers up to several inches away from the needle (Langevin et al., 2004). Increasing the amount of rotation also facilitates a linear increase in the amount of tissue displacement during subsequent axial needle rotation (Langevin et al., 2004), producing viscoelastic relaxation, flattening of the fibroblasts, and remodeling of the cytoskeleton (Langevin et al., 2011).

It is important also to state here that you must ensure that you have a thorough working knowledge of current safety guidelines (such as when and how to needle the thorax), contraindications, anatomical considerations (lung fields, arteries, nerves), hygiene guidelines, glove usage, and needle-disposal guidelines, and an excellent knowledge of anatomy prior to beginning your DN training.

For more information, I highly recommend *Trigger Point Dry Needling: An Evidence and Clinical-Based Approach* (Dommerholt and Fernandez-de-las-Penas, 2013).

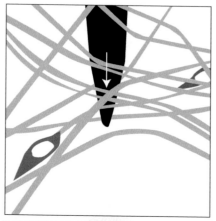

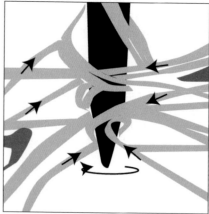

Figure 3.1: The "winding-up" effect of twiddling a needle

---

2. Allodynia is a pain due to a stimulus that does not normally provoke pain.

3. Hyperalgesia is an increased sensitivity to pain, which may be caused by damage to nociceptors or peripheral nerves.

References

Bron C, Dommerholtz J and Stegenga B (2011) High prevalence of shoulder girdle muscles with myofascial trigger points in patients with shoulder pain. *BMC Medicine* 9: 8

Chen Q, Bensamoun S, Basford JR, Thompson JN and An KN (2007) Identification and quantification of myofascial taut bands with magnetic resonance elastography. *Archives of Physical Medicine and Rehabilitation* 88(12): 1658–1661

Dommerholt J (2011) Dry needling: peripheral and central considerations. *Journal of Manipulative Therapy* 19(4): 223–227

Dommerholt J and Fernandez-de-las-Penas C (2013) *Trigger Point Dry Needling: An Evidence and Clinical Based Approach.* Oxford: Churchill Livingstone

Findley TW (2012) Fascia science and clinical applications: a clinician/researcher's perspectives. *Journal of Bodywork and Movement Therapies* 16(4): 67–75

Freeman MD, Nystrom A and Centeno C (2009) Chronic whiplash and central sensitisation; an evaluation of the role of a myofascial trigger point in pain modulation. *Journal of Brachial Plexus and Peripheral Nerve Injury* 4(1): 2

Gautam M, Benson CJ and Sluka KA (2010) Increased response of muscle sensory neurons to decreases in pH after muscle inflammation. *Neuroscience* 170: 893–900

Ge HY and Arendt-Nielsen L (2011) Latent myofascial trigger points. *Current Pain and Headache Reports* 15(5): 386–392

Ge HY, Zhang Y, Boudreau S, Yue SW and Arendt-Nielsen L (2008) Induction of muscle cramps by nociceptive stimulation of latent myofascial trigger points. *Experimental Brain Research* 187(4): 623–629

Gerwin RD (2008) The taut band and other mysteries of the trigger point: an examination of the mechanisms relevant to the development and maintenance of the trigger point. *Journal of Musculoskeletal Pain* 16: 115–121

Gerwin RD and Dommerholt J (2006) Treatment of myofascial pain syndromes. In: Boswell MV and Cole BE (eds) *Weiner's Pain Management, a Practical Guide for Clinicians.* Boca Raton, Florida: CRC Press

Hidalgo-Lozano A, Fernandez-de-las-Penas C, Alonso-Blanco C, Ge HY, Arendt-Nielsen L and Arroyo-Morales M (2010) Muscle trigger points and pressure pain hyperalgesia in the shoulder muscles in patients with unilateral shoulder impingement: a blinded, controlled study. *Experimental Brain Research* 202: 915–925

Hodges PW and Tucker K (2011) Moving differently in pain: a new theory to explain the adaptation of pain. *Pain* 152(3): S90–S98

Hoyle JA, Marras WS, Sheedy JE and Hart DE (2011) Effects of postural and visual stressors on myofascial trigger point development and motor unit rotation during computer work. *Journal of Electromyography and Kinesiology* 21(1): 41–48

Huang W, Pach D, Napadow V, Park K, Long X, Neurmann J, Maeda Y, Nierhaus T, Liang F and Witt CM (2012) Characterising acupuncture stimuli using brain imaging with FMR: a systematic review and meta-analysis of the literature. *Deutsche Zeitschrift für Akupunktur* 55(3): 26–28

Langevin HM, Bouffard NA and Fox JR (2011) Fibroblast cytoskeletal remodelling contributes to connective tissue tension. *Journal of Cellular Physiology* 226: 1166–1175

Langevin HM, Churchill DL and Cipolla MJ (2001) Mechanical signalling through connective tissue: a mechanism for the therapeutic effect of acupuncture. *FASEB Journal* 15(12): 2275–2282

Langevin HM, Churchill DL and Wu J (2002) Evidence of connective tissue involvement in acupuncture. *FASEB Journal* 16: 872–874

Langevin HM and Huijing PA (2009) Communicating about fascia: history, pitfalls, and recommendations. *International Journal of Therapeutic Massage and Bodywork* 2: 3–8

Langevin HM, Konofagou EE and Badger GJ (2004) Tissue displacements during acupuncture using ultrasound elastography techniques. *Ultrasound Medical Biology* 30: 1173–1183

Lucas KR, Polus BI and Rich PS (2004) Latent myofascial trigger points: their effects on muscle activation and movement efficiency. *Journal of Bodywork and Movement Therapies* 8(3): 160–166

Lucas KR, Rich PA and Polus BI (2010) Muscle activation patterns in the scapular positioning muscles during loaded scapular plane elevation: the effects of latent myofascial trigger points. *Clinical Biomechanics* 25: 765–770

McGrath S and White P (2015) The Role of Acupuncture in Neuropathic Pain Management: An Extended Literature Review. Unpublished MSc Literature Review, University of Southampton.

Melzack R (2001) Pain and the neuromatrix in the brain. *Journal of Dental Education* 65(12): 1378–1382

Mense S and Gerwin RD (2010) *Muscle Pain: Understanding the Mechanisms.* Berlin: Springer-Verlag

Moseley GL (2003) A pain neuromatrix approach to patients with chronic pain. *Manual Therapy* 8(3): 130–140

Moseley GL (2012) Teaching people about pain: why do we keep beating around the bush? *Pain Management* 2(1): 1–3

Napadow V, Kettner N, Lui J, Li M, Kwong KK, Vangel M, Makris N, Audette J and Hui KK (2007) Hypothalamus and amygdala response to acupuncture stimuli in carpal tunnel syndrome. *Pain* 130(3): 254–266

Nijs J, van Houdenhove B and Oostendorp RA (2010) Recognition of central sensitisation in patients with musculoskeletal pain: application of pain neurophysiology in manual therapy practice. *Manual Therapy* 15(2): 135–141

Puentedura EL and Louw A (2012) A neuroscience approach to managing athletes with low back pain. *Physical Therapy in Sport* 13(3): 123–133

Rha DW, Shin JC, Kim YK, Jung JH, Kim YU and Lee SC (2011) Detecting local twitch responses of myofascial trigger points in the lower back muscles using ultrasonography. *Archives of Physical Medicine and Rehabilitation* 92(10): 1576–1580

Simons DG and Mense S (1998) Understanding and measurement of muscle tone as related to clinical muscle pain. *Pain* 75(1): 1–17

Simons DG, Travell JG and Simons LS (1999) *Myofascial Pain and Dysfunction: The Trigger Point Manual*. Baltimore: Williams and Wilkins

Treaster D, Marras WS, Burr D, Sheedy J and Hart D (2006) Myofascial trigger point development form visual and postural stressors during computer work. *Journal of Electromyography and Kinesiology* 16(2): 115–124

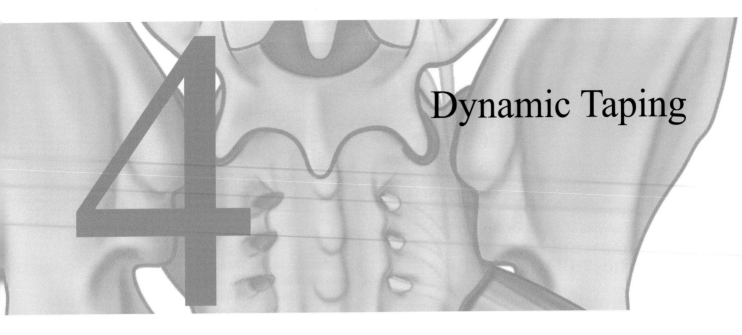

Dynamic Taping

Text written and supplied with thanks by Ryan Kendrick, Dynamic Tape®

Historically, taping approaches have been aimed at modifying movement patterns (arthrokinematics) or producing accessory motions (throughout the performance of a physiological motion), for example:

- Restricting plantar flexion and inversion to manage or prevent lateral ankle sprain (Trégouët et al., 2013)
- Resisting lateral translation of the patella in the management of patellofemoral pain syndrome (McConnell, 1996; Lee and Cho, 2013)
- The Mulligan approach (Mau and Baker, 2014; Yoon et al., 2014).

Support within the literature is dependent upon numerous factors (body region, technique, clinical condition, pathological stage, outcome measures). Moderate evidence is available (O'Sullivan et al., 2008; Franettovich et al., 2010; Maguire et al., 2010; Lee and Cho, 2013; Trégouët et al., 2013; Shaheen et al., 2014) supporting the role of rigid tapes when addressing electromyograph (EMG) modification and restricting range of movement (ROM). Very recently, support for the use of elastic bandaging and kinesiology tape has emerged (Cornwall et al., 2013; Song et al., 2014).

A number of studies (Vicenzino et al., 1997; Harradine et al., 2001; Noland and Kennedy, 2009) have looked at the integrity of rigid taping (tape fatigue) following exercise and found that the immediate improvements obtained following taping were significantly reduced after exercise. More recently, it has been found that elastic tape may perform slightly better; however, this evidence is relatively weak (Abián-Vicén et al., 2009).

Aims of Dynamic Taping

Dynamic taping aims to reduce the eccentric demand on the musculotendinous unit (MTU). Taping in a specific way generates a deceleration force and stores elastic potential once deceleration is complete. The initiation of fiber shortening releases the energy back into the kinetic chain, assisting the transition into the concentric cycle.

Techniques aim to provide:

- A strong mechanical effect without limiting ROM
- Deceleration and therefore load absorption through range
- Modification to the work of muscle (active assistance, resistance against gravity) without affecting ROM
- Modification of movement patterns, introduction of accessory motions (similar to Mulligan or McConnell techniques), using the strong recoil force of the tape without limiting ROM
- Maintenance of these effects (over several days) following significant exercise challenges (reduced tape fatigue)
- Potential reductions in pain
- Potential effect on motor control, and the proprioceptive and lymphatic systems.

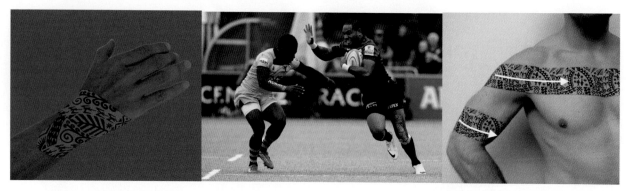

Figure 4.1: Examples of the various benefits of dynamic taping

Properties of Dynamic Tape®

- *Four-way stretching*: avoids limiting movement during complex tasks, especially when spiraling around limbs, crossing multiple joints, or taping across the midline; application of tapes crossing over one another will not reduce the recoil effect or limit ROM; reduction of skin traction (and therefore blisters); takes into consideration the pennation of muscles and may allow mimicking of the muscle action or provide multiple directional force simultaneously.

- *Strong resistance and recoil*: significant deceleration and active assistance; Powerband™ can be created by laminating two or more layers together prior to application.

- *High degree of stretch with no rigid end point*: applied with some resistance when muscle is shortened, creating tension as lengthening occurs; must be able to stretch over twice the original length without a rigid end point.

- *Reduces load*: when the tape is stretched quickly, more resistance is provided; correct application results in nonfatigue of the tape, reduced adverse effects, and longer wear time.

Biomechanical Principles

Levers

There are three classes of levers: first-, second-, and third-class. The class of lever is determined by the orientation of resistance and effort relative to the fulcrum (see Figures 4.2–4.4).

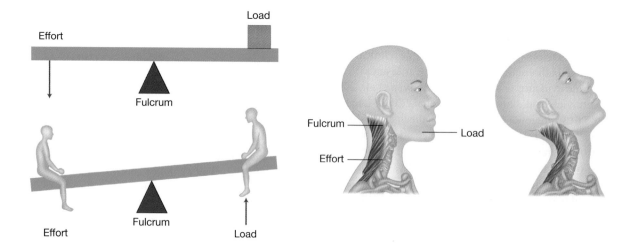

Figure 4.2: First-class lever: the relative position of the components is load-fulcrum-effort. Examples are a seesaw and a pair of scissors. In the body, an example is the ability to extend the head and neck: here the facial structures are the load, the atlanto-occipital joint is the fulcrum, and the posterior neck muscles provide the effort

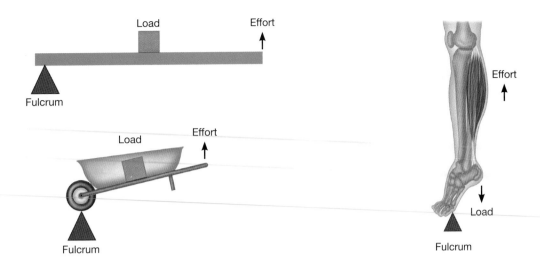

Figure 4.3: Second-class lever: the relative position of components is fulcrum-load-effort. The best example is a wheelbarrow. In the body, an example is the ability to raise the heels off the ground in standing: here the ball of the foot is the fulcrum, the body weight is the load, and the calf muscles provide the effort. With second-class levers, speed and range of motion are sacrificed for strength

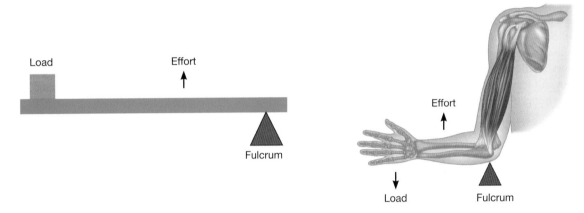

Figure 4.4: Third-class lever: the relative position of components is load-effort-fulcrum. A pair of tweezers is an example of this. In the body, most skeletal muscles act in this way. An example is flexing the forearm: here an object held in the hand is the load, the biceps provide the effort, and the elbow joint is the fulcrum. With third-class levers, strength is sacrificed for speed and range of motion

Influence of Muscle Length

All muscles have the ability to concentrically shorten, isometrically hold a position, and eccentrically lengthen, and in so doing, they all provide proprioception to the central nervous system. Muscles are most efficient and generate optimal force when they operate in their midrange. They are inefficient and can appear functionally weak when they are required to function in a shortened or lengthened range relative to their normal or habitual length. A muscle's structure also affects its ability to generate force. Muscles with long levers are biomechanically very efficient in producing ROM. They are not particularly efficient at preventing excessive movement at the axis of the joint or in eccentric movements. Conversely, muscles with short levers are efficient at controlling the axis to limit excessive movement and therefore protect against overstrain.

Fundamentals of Dynamic Taping

To obtain a genuine mechanical effect, three conditions must be met. The taping technique must:

- Cross a joint or joints—If the tape is to have any direct mechanical effect on motion at a joint, it must cross that joint and attach to the levers on either side.
- Be applied in a short position—The tape must be applied in a short position and stretched to the onset of resistance, so that a deceleration force is imparted as soon as lengthening commences.
- Obtain good purchase on the levers—The tape must be able to adhere well and gain good purchase on the levers that it is attempting to affect. There is a lot of soft tissue present, and some body parts are more easily taped than others.

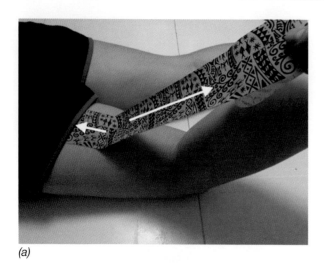
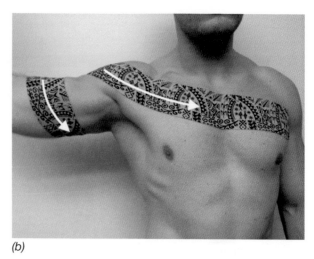

(a)   (b)

Figure 4.5: The fundamentals of dynamic taping: (a) across a joint or joints applied in a short position, (b) obtaining a good purchase on the levers, and using spiraling or split techniques

Spiraling or split techniques are often employed to take up the soft-tissue tension first and to gain good purchase on the lever. If this is not achieved, there is a lot of motion of the soft tissue but very little mechanical effect on the lever. Once again, a high degree of stretch is necessary to allow the soft-tissue tension to be taken up first but still leaving sufficient stretch and recoil to provide the bungee-like effect.

Mechanical Mechanisms

Professor David Sackett, who is credited as being a leader in the area of "evidence-based medicine," explains that the evidence available in the literature must be integrated and incorporated in the light of patient- and clinician-specific factors. The patient's wishes and expectations must be considered, and skillful assessment and diagnosis are required on the part of the clinician. Clinical experience and sound clinical reasoning must bridge the gap between what has been proven in research and the presenting patient, as there will never be research that is reliable, sensitive, and specific to each and every case. Only then can relevant interventions be considered and applied, if the risks are considered acceptable given the potential benefit. "If no randomized trial has been carried out for our patient's predicament, we must follow the trail to the next best external evidence and work from there" (Sackett et al., 1996).

Force Generation, and Energy Absorption, Storage, and Release

The applied tape extends well beyond the insertion of the muscle, thereby conferring a mechanical advantage. The tape's position on the skin places it further from the axis of rotation. As a result, the tape stretches further and faster than the musculotendinous unit (MTU) itself, absorbing and dissipating load and reducing the work and energy absorption requirements of the MTU. In addition, the elastic energy that is contributed in the outer range, when the tape is at maximum stretch, helps to compensate for the mechanical insufficiency of the muscle as determined by the length–tension relationship. The elastic recoil will reduce internal muscle force in early injury to allow movement without excessive load on the MTU (permitting a more functional healing response, reduction in compensatory strategies, and pain inhibition), through controlled loading.

Dynamic taping aims to reduce the load absorption requirements at the affected joint by providing some of the required force externally. Pain associated with tendinopathy is load dependent (more load = more pain). Load has been credited as being the driver that progresses tendinopathy (early reactive, disrepair, degenerative), but is essential for recovery; specific loading is critical (Cook and Purdham, 2009).

Augmentation of Force Closure

Panjabi (1992) describes stability in terms of the integration of three subsystems, the coordinated action of which permits effective or optimal load transfer across a joint. The three subsystems are the passive, active, and neural (neuromotor control) subsystems. The passive subsystem relates largely to the architecture of joints and passive restraining structures such as discs and ligaments, and is often referred to as "form closure." The active subsystem refers to the MTUs, which have an ability to apply force to the joint; this function is accordingly referred to as "force closure." The neural subsystem involves the central and peripheral nervous system and is responsible for timely and coordinated activation of muscles to maintain stability and efficiency within the system.

Panjabi also suggests that, to some extent, alteration in one system can be compensated for by one of the other systems.

Vleeming et al. (1992) demonstrated that a sacroiliac joint (SIJ) applied with fifty newtons of force is sufficient to significantly reduce sagittal sacral motion. They equated this force with the strength with which one ties a pair of shoelaces. Cholewicki et al. (1999) demonstrated that increasing intra-abdominal pressure and/or wearing an abdominal belt significantly increases spinal stability. Taping applications can be considered that may directly apply force across the SIJ or may provide firm support to the anterior abdominal wall to assist in development of intra-abdominal pressure.

Reducing Tissue Stress

De-loading tapes are commonly used in clinical practice and involve placing the target muscle and surrounding soft tissue in a shortened and relaxed position (manually gathering it or "pinching" it together) and then holding it in place with use of various taping techniques (McConnell, 2000). Hug et al. (2014) demonstrated that taping in this way results in a reduction in tissue stress (reducing stiffness within the tissues). This may have an impact on the compressive loading (shown to be a contributing factor in tendinopathy) and may also be beneficial when taping mechanosensitive neural tissue. Dynamic taping and the tape's elastic recoil properties create a very effective de-loading at the same time as permitting full range of motion.

Modifying Kinematics

Altered kinematics may be implicated in many injuries (Cornwall, 2000; Raissi et al., 2009; Ryan et al., 2009; Rathleff et al., 2012). This could be exacerbated by a number of factors, including faulty technique or equipment, weakness, inhibition, pain, training error, and inadequate recovery and adaptation periods. Dynamic taping may help to modify the altered kinematics mentioned (increasing stiffness of noncontractile elements, contributing to force generation, and improving the length–tension relationship of the muscle).

SIJ Points to Consider

- The SIJs are essential for effective load transfer between the spine and legs (Vleeming et al., 2012).
- SIJ dysfunction, pelvic-girdle pain, and ineffective load transfer have been termed SIJ incompetence (Cusi et al., 2013).
- Sacral nutation is associated with loaded positions, and counternutation with unloaded positions.
- Standing upright is generally associated with increased nutation (close-packed position), as are sitting and lying prone when compared with supine.
- Sacral nutation is essential for force closing the pelvis, and tightens most of the SIJ ligaments except the long dorsal ligament, which is tensioned by counternutation.
- Asymmetries have been demonstrated in pelvic-girdle pain, with counternutation occurring on the affected side (Mens et al., 1999; Hungerford et al., 2003).
- Muscle activity can contribute to force closure, especially the gluteus maximus, erector spinae, biceps femoris, transversus abdominis, and obliquus internus (Richardson et al., 2002; van Wingerden et al., 2004).
- Altered muscle activity has been demonstrated in pelvic-girdle pain populations including (Hungerford et al., 2003):
- *Gluteus maximus—delays, weakness, and increased activity ipsilaterally*
- *Obliquus internus—delays ipsilaterally*
- *Biceps femoris—activates sooner and increases activity*
- *Multifidus—delays ipsilaterally.*
- Metabolic disturbances with increased uptake demonstrated on SPECT-CT[1] imaging in dorsal SIJ ligaments, biceps femoris, and adductors (Cusi et al., 2013) suggest abnormal load, and combined with EMG studies may be suggestive of an attempt to generate sufficient tension to restore competence via the musculotendinous/ligamentous connections and in response to counternutation.
- External pelvic compression decreases laxity of the SIJ, changes lumbopelvic kinematics, alters selective recruitment of stabilizing musculature (including decreasing reaction time in gluteus maximus, increasing reaction time in biceps femoris, reducing overactivity of biceps femoris) (Jung et al., 2012), and reduces pain (Arumugam et al., 2012).

---

1. An imaging modality where a single-photon emission computed tomography image is merged or fused with a computed tomography image.

Physiological Mechanisms

Pain Physiology

Research and clinical observation state that the level of pain an individual may experience is not in direct proportion to the extent of tissue damage. Minor injuries can result in chronic, debilitating pain and severe injuries can recover completely, with much lower levels of pain (Beecher, 1946, 1955, 1960). Biochemical and neurogenic contributions are reported in the literature and good evidence is emerging to suggest that non-opioid-mediated hypoalgesia occurs following some manual therapy techniques (Abbott et al., 2001; Paungmali et al., 2004; Milner et al., 2006; Vicenzino et al., 2007; Franettovich et al., 2008; van Wilgen and Keizer, 2011).

How is Pain Perceived?

Pain receptors (nociceptors) send signals to certain areas of the spinal cord. These messages may be acted upon at this level, to either dampen them down or ramp them up. The signals then travel along nerves in the spinal cord to the brain, where they essentially pass through a number of filters, or are weighed up against a number of factors. These include, but are not limited to, factors such as beliefs, expectations, past experiences, social contexts, and environment, giving information regarding perceived threat (Moseley, 2007).

The outcome of this process or analysis will determine the degree of pain experienced. In other words, pain is not simply a sensory input but rather one output resulting from a complex process (Moseley, 2007). Putting this into context, a very recent study looking at sham surgery for osteoarthritis of the knee showed it to be as effective as the actual procedure (Moseley et al., 2002). If people believe that they will receive a less noxious stimulus, they generally report less pain than if they are told that they are going to receive a more painful stimulus, even though the stimuli administered are actually the same.

In some chronic pain states, pain is considered to be centrally mediated. Changes occurring at the spinal cord level (e.g. loss of inhibitory interneurons) and above can amplify the pain (hyperalgesia). Similarly, nerve fibers normally responsible for touch and pressure (mechanoreceptors) can grow into the area of the spinal cord normally occupied by nociceptive fibers. Conversion of nociceptors into wide dynamic neurons then occurs. Consequently, stimulation of the mechanoreceptors by touch or pressure can be transmitted up the spinal cord as if it had originated from a nociceptive fiber, and therefore normal light touch can be experienced as pain (Latremoliere and Woolf, 2009).

How Might Dynamic Taping Influence Pain?

The application of Dynamic Tape® could influence the pain pathways in a number of ways. Contributing to force generation (described above), the Dynamic Tape® may effectively reduce the load on injured tissue and therefore reduce the stimulation of sensitized nociceptors. Similarly, the de-loading aspect has been shown to reduce tissue stress or tension, which may also reduce stimulation of sensitized structures.

Dynamic Tape® can be applied in such a way as to shorten the damaged tissues in a similar way, but utilizing the elastic recoil of the tape to maximize the "boxing" of the soft tissue. This may help to approximate the torn ends of muscle fibers to aid healing, as well as to reduce the firing of nociceptors. Further, indirect support for this hypothesis is emerging with research demonstrating an immediate increase in pressure-pain thresholds following the application of strain–counterstrain techniques (Lewis et al., 2010), where the aim is to shorten the target tissue to a point where it is not registering as being under strain and then slowly return it to its resting position.

In addition to reducing mechanical stimulation of nociceptors, the tape may also induce a similar form of (non-opioid) hypoalgesia as has been demonstrated with other manual therapy techniques (Abbott et al., 2001; Paungmali et al. 2004; Vicenzino et al., 2007). Autonomic changes are often observed and further research is required to determine if a direct effect of this nature exists.

Melzack and Wall's gate control theory of pain suggests that stimulation of large-diameter mechanoreceptors can "close the gate," or flood the ascending pathways, thereby reducing the transmission of pain signals (Melzack and Wall, 1965). The constant and varying stimulation of dynamic taping may stimulate the large-diameter fibers to reduce the transmission of painful stimuli.

If an athlete has strong beliefs or positive previous experiences with tape it is likely that it will have a positive effect in managing his or her pain and tissue healing.

Using Dynamic Tape®

Adverse Reactions

There are generally three common types of reaction that occur with all adhesive tapes. The adhesive used on Dynamic Tape® has been tested and rated as non-sensitizing, non-irritating, and nontoxic, and is considered a very low allergy tape.

The three reaction types most likely to occur with any adhesive tape include:

1. Allergic Reaction

This is a severe contact dermatitis.

Allergic reactions will:

- Happen quickly—usually within fifteen to thirty minutes
- Be irritated all over, anywhere that has been covered with tape
- Get hot and itchy
- Cause red, raised skin and welts if left too long.

WARNINGS must be given to **ALL** patients and the tape **MUST** be removed immediately should any signs of allergic reaction appear (heat, itching, burning, stinging, irritation, or redness). Failure to remove the tape can result in extremely nasty reactions. The reaction above occurred when a tape was left in situ for two days despite signs of allergic reaction commencing after a short period.

DO NOT tell people that they **MUST** keep it on for a certain period of time. If all is going well and it is not causing irritation, they may leave it on for up to five days.

2. Contact Dermatitis

This generally occurs with the cotton-based products that become moist and remain in contact with the skin for several days. These do not generally occur with Dynamic Tape® owing to the fabric being breathable and quick drying.

3. Mechanical Irritation

This can occur with any tape if excessive tension or shearing on the skin occurs. Owing to the energy contained within Dynamic Tape® and the way in which it is used, this can occur if the "Directions for Use" are not followed. Mechanical reactions generally occur in the form of traction blisters.

Traction blisters will:

- Occur at isolated points on the tape—usually at the ends
- Commence after about ten hours (may be sooner) up to a few days, depending on the amount of tension on the skin
- Commence by stinging, burning, or itching or just a very sensitive feeling under the end of the tape.

If the tape is removed when these symptoms occur, usually a little redness is all that results. Blisters should **NOT** occur. If the patient has been **WARNED** appropriately, **UNDERSTOOD** this warning, and **COMPLIED** with these directions, he or she will remove the tape before a blister results.

These can and do occur if too much tension is present and the patient is not properly warned or ignores this warning. It is user error and not an allergic reaction to the tape. They are easy to avoid if the application guidelines are adhered to.

Directions for Use

Dynamic taping is not a "cookbook" approach. Techniques are developed and applied according to assessment findings, treatment approach, and patient goals. Condition-based techniques—e.g. taping every back pain or every patellar tendinopathy in the same way—yield average results. Standardized techniques may be useful as a guideline but fail to recognize the importance of identifying key contributing factors, which can then be the focus of the taping application.

The techniques demonstrated in this book, therefore, serve only as an example of how clinical reasoning can be combined with the current evidence to develop an appropriate technique.

It is important to know how to apply the tape correctly to get optimal adhesion and to reduce the risk of adverse reactions. If adverse reactions occur, it is important to be able to differentiate between allergic reactions, which happen rarely, and a mechanical irritation, which happen often owing to faulty technique (but should not happen at all).

The adhesive on Dynamic Tape® is stronger than that on most tapes and should therefore adhere well if applied correctly. It is, however, designed to lift away if too much tension is applied, to reduce the risk of traction blisters.

Important Considerations

- Prepare the skin correctly.
- Remove the backing sheet by tearing the paper so that fingers do not come into contact with the adhesive.
- Leave adequate anchor points with no tension—three to four fingers' width.
- Anchor the tape at a point three to four fingers' width away from the end, then apply gentle tension to the skin in the opposite direction so that tension is not transmitted to the skin—this will also remove any skin creases from under the tape.
- Only tension the tape to the very onset of resistance. This is almost immediate. Do not stretch strongly. Familiarize yourself with the Dynamic Tape®. Practice gently stretching the tape until you have a good appreciation of the point at which the resistance commences.

Developing Techniques

Dynamic taping is dependent upon a sound clinical reasoning process and treatment approach. The biomechanical rationale therefore dictates that dynamic taping is fluid and evolving rather than rigid or prescriptive. Manual therapists the world over draw on different skills and expertise to address their clients' conditions, the clients and conditions themselves also exhibiting a large degree of heterogeneity. A rigorous assessment and thorough consideration of the functional anatomy and biomechanics displayed will allow an appropriate dynamic taping application to be developed to complement other treatment modalities.

The most critical element in maximizing the effect of your dynamic taping technique is a sound rationale and clearly defined aim of the intervention. A primary hypothesis must be formulated from thorough subjective and physical examination, interpreted against a background of pathology, pathoanatomy, pathophysiology, and pathomechanics.

Questioning regarding the history, site, nature, and irritability of symptoms, along with aggravating and easing factors, can help to identify potential causes and contributing factors and direct the physical examination. The physical examination should be designed to disprove the primary hypothesis and exclude the potential causes in order to prevent a confirmation bias (only testing factors that confirm the primary hypothesis or omitting or dismissing evidence to the contrary).

In some cases this process will evolve over a couple of treatment sessions as the contribution of various factors is dissected out. Taping, both dynamic and rigid, can assist in assessment as well as treatment. Tape can be quickly applied to test a hypothesis and results can often be gleaned quickly—i.e. an immediate change in gait pattern and concurrent reduction in symptoms. Although this does not necessarily confirm cause and effect, it provides support for the primary hypothesis.

The assessment should implicate the structure or structures involved (there is rarely only one, particularly in longstanding conditions). These may be articular, myofascial, or neural structures. It should provide insight into the type of injury, the stage of pathology, and the pain processes at play. Contributing factors such as training, equipment, or biomechanical errors should be identified.

From this analysis we can determine what positions or movements may be aggravating the condition or, as is often overlooked, easing the condition—e.g. a simple rotation glide at the thumb may permit full, pain-free opposition in an otherwise painfully limited condition. It may be identified that the patient is holding the limb in an antalgic position to reduce excursion of painfully mechanosensitized neural tissue, e.g. in a radiculopathy. It may be as simple as determining that the patient has sprained the anterior talofibular ligament and that plantar flexion and inversion should be avoided to reduce load on this structure. A patient may present with a foot drop and is catching the toe during gait. Assistance to maintain more dorsiflexion would be advantageous.

Axis of Rotation

Once you have determined whether you are assisting muscle function, modifying the movement pattern, offloading a nerve, controlling joint motion, or addressing some other issue, the next step is to determine where the movement is occurring. The axis of rotation, line of pull, and position are all intimately related. Identifying these correctly will allow optimal techniques to be developed. Small changes can result in an effect opposite to the desired one.

The axis of rotation is generally readily identified with movements involving the large joints and with gross movements of the limbs and spine. Simply ask, "Where is the movement occurring?" Do not forget that there may be a rotation component or that multiple joints and movements may be involved. For example, a technique to reduce load on the long head of the biceps brachii tendon may involve resisting elbow extension (assist eccentric lowering) and then recoil back to assist elbow flexion (it is believed that Dynamic Tape® probably has more effect during the eccentric phase as the tape is lengthening and tensioning and is well positioned to absorb load and decelerate movement). Biceps brachii, however, has multiple functions and is influenced by other factors. A better technique may also contribute to supination, weight relief of the upper limb, resisting anterior translation of the humeral head and assisting upward rotation and control of the scapula. This clearly involves movement at several joints or several fulcrum points and multiple planes of movement.

Line of Pull

The line of pull relative to the axis of rotation will determine the direction of force introduced into the system. This must be consistent with your aim.

Force Vectors

When Dynamic Tape® is stretched either during application or through movement of the body part, it stores energy as elastic potential energy roughly equal to the amount of energy that was used to stretch it in the first place (as the tape is viscoelastic, a small amount of energy may be lost). The tape is often applied to use momentum to create the stretch; resistance and a deceleration force follow so that no active muscle work is required to tension the tape. In this way it will aid an eccentric muscle contraction, which is also working to decelerate the limb or control lengthening of the musculotendinous unit. The stored elastic potential energy will then be converted to kinetic energy as shortening occurs.

The direction of the tape will allow multiple effects from one piece of tape (see Figure 4.6a). Any vector can be broken down into its component vectors (gray). In other words, a vector in the northwesterly direction consists of a westerly vector and a northerly vector.

Consideration should be given to all vector directions as determined by the line of pull as these can be extremely clinically relevant.

When adding vectors, they must be added head to tail, and the light gray arrow in Figure 4.6b represents this. The resultant vector is in a medial and superior direction. In addition, as the tape is anterior to the axis of the tibiofemoral joint, it will tension as the knee flexes and this increased tension will not only resist lateral translation more but will also resist knee flexion, thereby assisting the eccentric action of the quadriceps mechanism. It is therefore essential to start and finish the tape medially to create resistance to lateral translation. It is also essential to ensure that the tape hooks in around the lateral border of the patella in order to provide mechanical resistance. Soft-tissue contours, genu recurvatum, and other factors may reduce the ability to get sufficient purchase on the patella in some people.

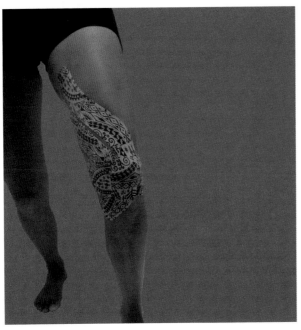
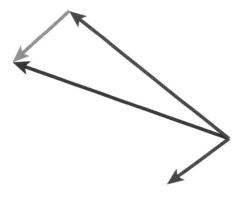

Figure 4.6: (a) Patellofemoral lateral sling. (b) Force diagram. The two dark gray arrows represent the direction of pull of the tape exerted on the lateral aspect of the patella toward the two anchor points at the end of the tape. The patella is acting like a stone in a slingshot

The concept of vector summation is also a fundamental tenet of the dynamic taping approach. If a certain amount of force is required to decelerate the limb and some of that force can be provided externally through the resistance of the tape, less intrinsic force is required by the body.

Position

The elastic energy within the Dynamic Tape® can only be effectively utilized if the tape is applied in the correct position. If the tape is too long (applied at the end of range) the tape will not resist the motion, nor will any elastic potential energy be stored at the end of range.

Dynamic Tape® must be applied (with the musculotendinous unit, joint, nerve) in the relatively shortened position. However, it is necessary to determine where in range the resistance should commence (e.g. for hamstring application prior to kicking a ball, if the tape is applied in ninety degrees of knee flexion, it will start to stretch and resist when the player is still generating force with the quadriceps). The aim would be to have the tape resisting and decelerating motion in terminal extension when the quadriceps is inactive and the hamstring is working eccentrically to control the follow through at the hip and knee. It is therefore recommended that the Dynamic Tape® be applied in about forty-five degrees from full extension with minimal stretch.

Leverage

When applying Dynamic Tape® do not simply copy the anatomy of the muscles. Many of the muscles have short lever arms or are class-three levers and therefore have an inherent mechanical disadvantage. It is possible to compensate for this to some degree by ensuring that we have a longer lever arm with the Dynamic Tape®. By starting the tape further from the fulcrum or axis of rotation we exert our force further down the limb and create a longer lever arm. If we use a longer crow bar, we can shift a greater resistance/load by using the same amount of force. The same holds true with the tape. Exerting the force further away from the fulcrum will result in greater torque production.

Furthermore, the tape will stretch further and sooner than the musculotendinous unit itself and therefore will begin to resist and decelerate motion. It also allows room for a large anchor point, which will improve adhesion and reduce the likelihood of mechanical irritation to the skin.

Evaluation

Always evaluate the effectiveness of the technique. Has it achieved the aims set out at the beginning?

- Ask the patient what they are feeling.
- Observe the changes in motion. Have you created the desired effect?
- Test and retest—always test pre- and post-taping.

In most cases an immediate effect is obtained. Sometimes the reduction in loading (twenty-four hours per day over several days) provides the effect, when an immediate change during objective reassessment is not observed. Even in these cases, subjectively the patient generally reports that it feels much better with the tape on. Reassessment will be more important between sessions rather than within a session in this instance.

By applying these principles, dynamic taping techniques become effective, specific, and targeted, and complement evidenced-based interventions.

For more information on dynamic taping, see: *www.dynamictape.info*

References

Abbott JH, Patla CE, and Jensen RH (2001) The initial effects of an elbow mobilization with movement technique on grip strength in subjects with lateral epicondylalgia. *Manual Therapy* 6(3): 163–169

Abián-Vicén J, Alegre LM, Fernández-Rodríguez JM, and Aguado X (2009) Prophylactic ankle taping: elastic versus inelastic taping. *Foot and Ankle International* 30(3): 218–225

Arumugam A, Milosavljevic S, Woodley S, and Sole G (2012) Effects of external pelvic compression on form closure, force closure, and neuromotor control of the lumbopelvic spine: a systematic review. *Manual Therapy* 17(4): 275–284; doi: 10.1016/j.math.2012.01.010. [Epub ahead of print, 2 March 2012]

Beecher HK (1946) Pain in men wounded in battle. *Annals of Surgery*, 123(1): 96–105

Beecher HK (1955) The powerful placebo. *JAMA* 159(17): 1602–1606

Beecher HK (1960) Control of suffering in severe trauma: usefulness of a quantitative approach. *JAMA* 173: 534–536

Cholewicki J, Juluru K, Radebold A, Panjabi MM, and McGill SM (1999) Lumbar spine stability can be augmented with an abdominal belt and/or increased intra-abdominal pressure. *European Spine Journal* 8(5): 388–395

Cook JL and Purdham CR (2009) Is tendinopathy a continuum: a pathology model to explain the clinical presentation of load-induced tendinopathy. *British Journal of Sports Medicine* 43: 409–416

Cornwall MW (2000) Common pathomechanics of the foot. *Athletic Therapy Today* 5(1): 10–16

Cornwall MW, Lebec M, DeGeyter J, and McPoil TG (2013). The reliability of the modified reverse-6 taping procedure with elastic tape to alter the height and width of the medial longitudinal arch. *International Journal of Sports Physical Therapy* 8(4): 381–392

Cusi M, Saunders J, van der Wall H, and Fogelman I (2013) Metabolic disturbances identified by SPECT-CT in patients with a clinical diagnosis of sacroiliac joint incompetence. *European Spine Journal* 22(7): 1674–1682; doi 10.1007/s00586-013-2725-5

Franettovich M, Chapman A, Blanch P, and Vicenzino B (2008) A physiological and psychological basis for anti-pronation taping from a critical review of the literature. *Sports Medicine* 38: 617–631

Franettovich M, Chapman AR, Blanch P, and Vicenzino B (2010) Augmented low-Dye tape alters foot mobility and neuromotor control of gait in individuals with and without exercise-related leg pain. *Journal of Foot and Ankle Research* 3: 5

Harradine P, Herrington L, and Wright R (2001) The effect of Low Dye taping upon rear-foot motion and position before and after exercise. *Foot* (Edinburgh, Scotland) 11: 57–60

Hug F, Ouellette A, Vicenzino B, Hodges PW, and Tucker K (2014) Deloading tape reduces muscle stress at rest and during contraction. *Medicine and Science in Sports and Exercise* 46(12): 2317–2325. [Epub ahead of print 28 April 2014]

Hungerford B, Gilleard W, and Hodges P (2003) Evidence of altered lumbopelvic muscle recruitment in the presence of sacroiliac joint pain. *Spine* 28: 1593–1600

Jung HS, Jeon HS, Oh DW, and Kwon OY (2012) Effect of the pelvic compression belt on the hip extensor activation patterns of sacroiliac joint pain patients during one-leg standing: a pilot study. *Manual Therapy* 18(2): 143–148; doi: 10.1016/j.math.2012.09.003. [Epub ahead of print, 27 October 2012]

Kendrick R (2013a) *Dynamic Taping Advanced Guide.* Posture Pals Pty Ltd.

Kendrick R (2013b) *Dynamic Taping Quick Start Guide.* PosturePals Pty Ltd.

Latremoliere A and Woolf C (2009) Central sensitisation: a generator of pain hypersensitivity by central neural plasticity. *Journal of Pain* 10(9): 895–926

Lee S-E and Cho S-H (2013) The effect of McConnell taping on vastus medialis and lateralis activity during squatting in adults with patellofemoral pain syndrome. *Journal of Exercise Rehabilitation* 9(2): 326–330

Lewis C, Khan A, Souvlis T, and Sterling M (2010) A randomised controlled study on the short term effects of strain-counterstrain treatment on quantitative sensory measures at digitally tender points in the low back. *Manual Therapy* 15(6): 536–541

Maguire C, Sieben JM, Frank M, and Romkes J (2010) Hip abductor control in walking following stroke: the immediate effect of canes, taping and TheraTogs on gait. *Clinical Rehabilitation* 24(1): 37–45

Mau H and Baker RT (2014) A modified mobilization-with-movement to treat a lateral ankle sprain. *International Journal of Sports Physical Therapy* 9(4): 540–548

McConnell J (1996) Management of patellofemoral problems. *Manual Therapy* 1: 6096e

McConnell J (2000) A novel approach to pain relief pre-therapeutic exercise. *Journal of Science and Medicine in Sport* 3: 325–334

Melzack R and Wall PD (1965) Pain mechanisms: a new theory. *Science* 150(3699): 971–979

Mens JM, Vleeming A, Snijders CJ, Stam HJ, and Ginai AZ (1999) The active straight leg raising test and mobility of the pelvic joints. *European Spine Journal* 8, 468–473

Milner CE, Ferber R, Pollard CD, Hamill J, and Davis IS (2006) Biochemical factors associated with tibial stress fracture in female runners. *Medicine and Science in Sports and Exercise* 38(2): 323–328

Moseley GL (2007) Reconceptualising pain according to modern pain science. *Physical Therapy Reviews* 12(3): 169–178

Moseley JB, O'Malley K, Petersen NJ, Menke TJ, Brody BA, Kuykendall DH, Hollingsworth JC, Ashton CM, and Wray NP (2002) A controlled trial of arthroscopic surgery for osteoarthritis of the knee. *New England Journal of Medicine* 347(2): 81–88

Nolan D and Kennedy N (2009) Effects of low-dye taping on plantar pressure pre and post exercise: an exploratory study. *BMC Musculoskeletal Disorders* 10: 40

O'Sullivan K, Kennedy N, O'Neill E, and Ni Mhainin U (2008) The effect of low-dye taping on rear-foot motion and plantar pressure during the stance phase of gait. *BMC Musculoskeletal Disorders* 9: 111

Panjabi MM (1992) The stabilizing system of the spine: Part I—function, dysfunction, adaptation, and enhancement. *Journal of Spinal Disorders and Techniques* 5(4): 383–389; discussion 397

Paungmali A, O'Leary S, Souvlis T, and Vincenzino B (2004) Naloxone fails to antagonize initial hypoalgesic effect of a manual therapy treatment for lateral epicondylalgia. *Journal of Manipulative and Physiological Therapeutics* 27(3): 180–185

Raissi GRD, Cherati ADS, Mansoori KD, and Razi MD (2009) The relationship between lower extremity alignment and medial tibial stress syndrome among non-professional athletes. *Sports Medicine, Arthroscopy, Rehabilitation, Therapy and Technology* 1: 11

Rathleff MS, Kelly LA, Christensen FB, Simonsen OH, Kaalund S, and Laessoe U (2012) Dynamic midfoot kinematics in subjects with medial tibial stress syndrome. *Journal of the American Podiatric Medical Association* 102(3): 205–212

Richardson CA, Snijders CJ, Hides JA, Damen L, Pas MS, and Storm J (2002) The relation between the transversus abdominis muscles, sacroiliac joint mechanics, and low back pain. *Spine* 27: 399–405

Ryan M, Grau S, Krauss I, Maiwald C, Taunton J, and Horstmann T (2009) Kinematic analysis of runners with Achilles mid-portion tendinopathy. *Foot and Ankle International* 30(12): 1190–1195

Sackett DL, Rosenberg WM, Gray JA, Haynes RB, and Richardson WS (1996) Evidence based medicine: what it is and what it isn't. *BMJ* (Clinical Research ed.) 312(7023): 71–72

Shaheen AF, Bull AM, and Alexander CM (2014) Rigid and elastic taping changes scapular kinematics and pain in subjects with shoulder impingement syndrome: an experimental study. *Journal of Electromyography and Kinesiology* 25(1): 84–92

Song CY, Huang HY, Chen SC, Lin JJ and Chang AH (2014) Effects of femoral rotational taping on pain, lower extremity kinematics, and muscle activation in female patients with patellofemoral pain. *Journal of Science and Medicine in Sport* 18(4): 388–393. [Epub ahead of print, 24 July 2014]

Trégouët P, Merland F, and Horodyski MB (2013) A comparison of the effects of ankle taping styles on biomechanics during ankle inversion. *Annals of Physical and Rehabilitation Medicine* 56(2): 113–122

van Wilgen CP and Keizer D (2011) Neuropathic pain mechanisms in patients with chronic sports injuries: a diagnostic model useful in sports medicine? *Pain Medicine* 12(1): 110–117

van Wingerden JP, Vleeming A, Buyruk HM, and Raissadat K (2004) Stabilization of the sacroiliac joint in vivo: verification of muscular contribution to force closure of the pelvis. *European Spine Journal* 13: 199–205

Vicenzino B, Cleland JA, and Bisset L (2007) Joint manipulation in the management of lateral epicondylalgia: a clinical commentary. *Journal of Manual and Manipulative Therapy* 15(1): 50–56

Vicenzino B, Feilding J, Howard R, Moore R, and Smith S (1997) An investigation of the antipronation effect of two taping methods after application and exercise. *Gait and Posture* 5(1): 1–5

Vleeming A, Buyruk HM, Stoeckart R, Karamursel S, and Snijders CJ (1992) An integrated therapy for peripartum pelvic instability: a study of the biomechanical effects of pelvic belts. *American Journal of Obstetrics and Gynecology* 166(4): 1243–1247

Vleeming A, Schuenke MD, Masi AT, Carreiro JE, Danneels L, and Willard FH (2012) The sacroiliac joint: an overview of its anatomy, function and potential clinical implications. *Journal of Anatomy* 221: 537–567

Yoon J, Hwang Y, An D, and Oh J (2014). Changes in kinetic, kinematic, and temporal parameters of walking in people with limited ankle dorsiflexion: pre-post application of modified mobilization with movement using talus glide taping. *Journal of Manipulative and Physiological Therapeutics* 37(5): 320–325

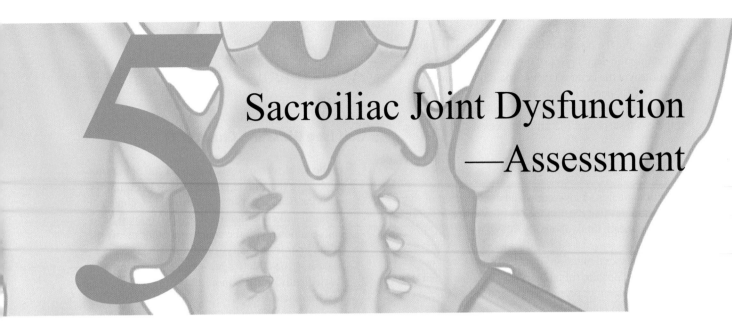

Sacroiliac Joint Dysfunction —Assessment

Altered biomechanics are deciphered by the body as a whole resulting in adaptive shortening and lengthening of associated structures. The body continues to make adaptations long after the initial injury, and this may be the reason why the athlete in front of you can't quite put his or her finger on when or how the presenting problem arose, leading to the subsequent label of "insidious onset."

The biomechanical adaptations following the initial insult/injury/illness often result in muscle imbalances, which by their very nature inhibit muscle activation or produce overactive or hypertonic muscles (also weak), taking the muscles into a position of being too long and dysfunctional or too short and dysfunctional. Depending on the load being placed on the body and the lines of stress attempting to control the structures (which are dysfunctional), this information will guide you toward your treatment goal. For example, the ligaments and fascia of the pelvis and sacrum (thoracolumbar and abdominal aponeurosis) may be loaded in unfamiliar patterns following injury to the spine, resulting in altered positions of the pelvis … and on it goes.

It is clear that the ilia and sacrum are at the center of sacroiliac dysfunction and pain, but what of the relationship between dysfunction of the sacroiliac joint (SIJ) and the hip joints' range of movement (ROM)? Without correct alignment of the femur and its articulation with the acetabulum, and fully functioning ROM, how is the pelvis able to absorb the forces of impact during walking, running, jumping, etc.? How do the structures crossing that joint adapt—with inhibition, facilitation, or spasm (Janda, 1992)? The primary function of the lumbopelvic-hip complex is to transfer loads safely while fulfilling the movement and control requirements of a task (Lee and Lee, 2010). Coexisting dysfunctions in the areas adjacent to the pelvis—such as movement disorders of the hip, lumbar spine, and neurodynamics—are also very common.

Considerations—Prior to Treatment

Before proceeding with any form of therapy (Rx) input it is important that all associated structures impacting on the injured/dysfunctional areas are assessed for their lack of, or excessive involvement in, the symptoms being presented to you by the athlete. In addition, a thorough examination and assessment of the lumbar spine and bilateral hips should have preceded the assessment of the pelvis.

You should ensure that you assess the length and power of the structures being presented to you in this book in order for you to have a form of "outcome measure" on which to base your therapeutic input.

1. Assess the relevant structures bilaterally for length and power.
   - Use an outcome measure (if appropriate).
2. Using your clinical reasoning (obtained from your subjective and objective findings) decide what your soft-tissue treatment/input will be.
3. Implement that input.
4. Reassess.
   - Using the outcome measure selected (if appropriate).
5. Have you made the change you were looking for?
   - No? Select another "tool" from your physical therapy "toolbox."
   - Reassess.
   - Yes? Stop, do not overwork the tissues.
6. Give the athlete a rehabilitative exercise to help maintain the work you have done.

For example, the posterior fibers of the internal oblique invest into the deep layers of the contralateral gluteus maximus via the central layer of the thoracolumbar fascia (TLF), performing as a stabilizer system for the SIJ in low-load activities (such as walking). Therefore, if there is a suspected SIJ problem, assess the obliques.

Palpation

Palpation creates an awareness and appreciation of the huge variables that exist in the people we treat. Before charging ahead, think about the following:

- Check sacral nutation[1] in static upright weight-bearing posture (nutation is not the same when the person is either prone or supine; this has a huge impact on leg length).
- Shifting of the trochanter following an ankle sprain or orthotics that do not fit well may contribute to force closure of the SIJ and counterrotation of the ilia, resulting in leg-length inequalities.
- Iliosacral obliquity can also create the illusion of leg-length discrepancy.

Leg-Length Assessment

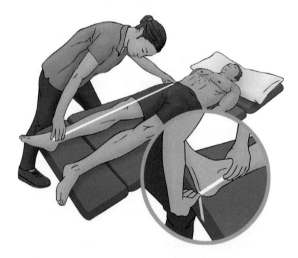

Figure 5.1: The process for assessing leg length. (1) The patient should be supine. (2) Measure from the anterior superior iliac spine (ASIS) to the medial malleolus (true leg length), then (3) extend the measurement down to the bottom of the heel with the ankle in neutral. (4) Assess before and after soft-tissue input and see if there is a change in your results (due to shortening of muscles acting on femur position). (5) True leg-length discrepancy—the patient may be in need of orthotics

Observation and Clearing Assessments—Prior to SIJ Assessment

Gait (see Glossary, Chapter 1)

1. In the ideal scenario you will have the opportunity to observe the athlete in all of his or her training sessions (walking, running, sprinting, technical, strength and conditioning (S&C)). You will have conversations with the coach and other members of the interdisciplinary/transprofessional team regarding the athlete's presenting symptoms.
2. Realistically, you are more likely to see that athlete in a treatment area.
3. Look closely at how the athlete walks into your treatment room; if this is not enough, have them walk up and down the hallway.
4. Observing how the athlete is loading through the pelvis and the lower extremities provides valuable information.
5. Expect to see good function:
   - No sign of Trendelenberg[2] gait
   - Good motor control
   - Alignment of lumbar spine, pelvis (with minimal rotation), and the joints below
   - Head and body producing fluid movement with minimal deviations laterally.
6. You may, however, see indications of failed load transfer:
   - Trendelenberg sign
   - Increased rotation of:
     - *Lumbar spine*
     - *Pelvis*
     - *Femur (medial rotation)*
     - *Foot (pronation)*
   - Increase in trunk deviation.
7. In addition, standing and sitting observations may include the following that may lead to tissue overload:
   - Increase in lumbar lordosis/swayback in standing
     - *Maximum sacral nutation*
     - *Symphysis pubis lying in front of the sternal notch*
   - Slumped sitting position
     - *Counternutation[3] of the sacrum.*

---

1. Nutation—flexion of the sacrum (see Glossary, Chapter 1).
2. Trendelenberg gait—the hip drops on the toe-off leg owing to weak abductors on the contralateral side (see Glossary, Chapter 1).
3. Sacral counternutation—extension of the sacrum (see Glossary, Chapter 1).

Clearing the Lumbar Spine (Lx)

1. *Lumbar flexion (figure 5.2)*
   - Therapist places two to three fingers on the lumbar vertebrae
   - Athlete flexes lumbar spine
   - Fingers should move apart
2. Whilst in lumbar flexion, add cervical flexion (dural, spinal cord tension)
3. *Lumbar extension (figure 5.3)*
   - Therapist places two to three fingers on the lumbar vertebrae
   - Athlete extends lumbar spine
   - Fingers should move closer together

4. *Athlete performs right- and left-side flexion (figure 5.4)*
5. *Athlete performs right and left lumbar quadrant (combined movements/multi-plane)—only do this if you have not yet provoked the symptoms in the previous clearing movements (figure 5.5)*
   - Quadrant test
     - *Extension*
     - *Side flexion*
     - *Right rotation/left rotation*
     - *Add overpressure[4] (stabilize the sacrum).*

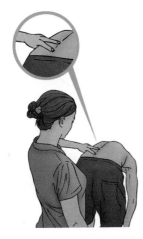

Figure 5.2: Lumbar-flexion assessment

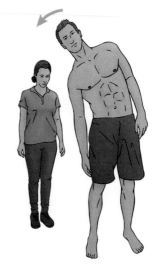

Figure 5.4: Lumbar-side-flexion assessment

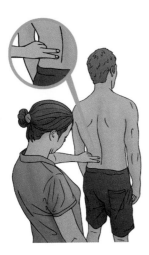

Figure 5.3: Lumbar-extension assessment

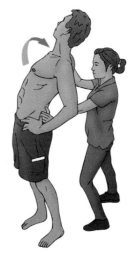

Figure 5.5: Quadrant assessment

4. Overpressure—passive end-of-range stretch without pain as a barrier.

Clearing the Hips

Assessing for Quantity and Quality of Movement

Any loss of range or quality of movement indicates hip involvement, which may be compensatory.

1. Athlete squats (body weight) with heels on and off the ground
    - Excessive lumbar flexion = there may be a hip-flexion restriction
2. Assess both sides for comparison
3. Full hip flexion in supine position with added overpressure (a)

4. Full internal rotation of the hip in supine position (reduction in range may indicate osteoarthritis) (b)
5. Follow immediately by full external rotation of the hip in supine position (c)
6. Full hip extension in prone position with added overpressure (d)
7. Full internal and external rotation of the hip in prone position (e and f).

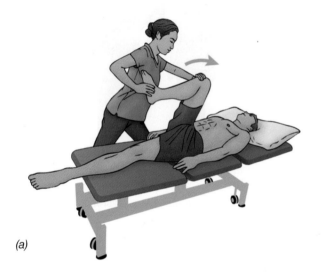

(a)

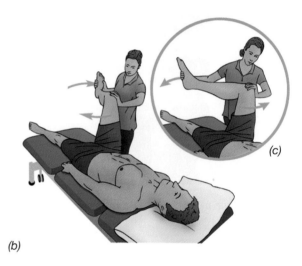

(b)

(c)

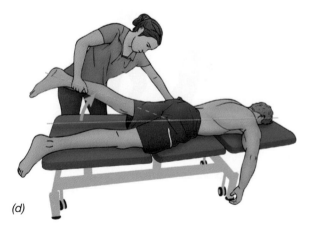

(d)

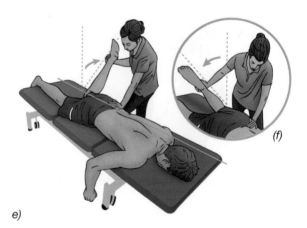

e)

(f)

Figure 5.6: Assessing for quantity and quality of movement

Neurodynamic Testing

Slump Test

The slump test assesses the whole nervous system but is most commonly known as the "lumbar neural tension test." The slump test:

1. Applies traction to the nerve roots by incorporating both spinal and hip flexion; pain provocation indicates nerve-root compression when the straight-leg raise (SLR) test is negative
2. Has been found to be more sensitive than the SLR in patients with lumbar disc herniation (Majlesi et al., 2008)
3. Can be uncomfortable and provocative—please ensure:
   - That you do not perform this test unless you have been taught the proper handling skills
   - That the subjective and objective findings indicate a slump test should be performed
   - All contraindications have been taken into account
   - That the ultimate aim of this test is to reproduce the athlete's symptoms
4. Is performed with the athlete seated on the edge of plinth
   - Hands clasped behind the back
   - Thoracic flexion closely followed by lumbar flexion
     - *Puts pressure on the lumbar discs*
   - Cervical flexion (with slight overpressure from therapist)
     - *Puts a stretch on the sciatic nerve*
   - Position is held as athlete extends one knee
   - Foot is then dorsiflexed
     - *Reproduction of pain anywhere from the lumbar spine to the foot is indicative of potential herniated disc, neural tension, or altered neurodynamics*
   - Cervical extension
     - *Pain disappears? Confirm findings by reducing neural tension*
   - Repeat other side and compare
5. Positive test
   - Reproduction of athlete's pain
6. Negative test
   - No pain
   - Discomfort in the leg due to normal muscle tightness.

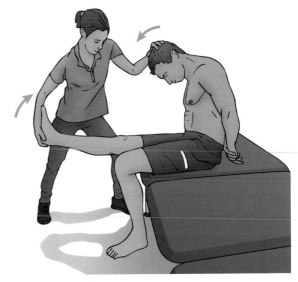

Figure 5.7: The slump test

Overhead Squat Assessment

In this assessment, the following are typically asymmetrical:

- Knee valgus (knees point toward the midline (knock knee))
- Knee varus (knees point outward, away from the midline (bow leg))
- Anterior pelvic tilt (a)
- Excessive lumbar flexion (b)
- Asymmetrical weight shift (indicative of SIJ dysfunction) (c)

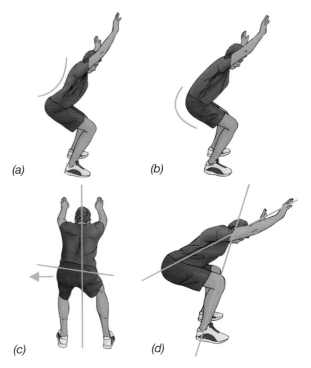

(a)   (b)

(c)   (d)

Figure 5.8: Overhead squat assessment

Ely's Test

The Ely's test is used to rule out rectus femoris as a source of anterior pelvis tilt.

1. Athlete prone and in alignment
   Therapist places finger and thumb of one hand on the posterior superior iliac spine (PSIS) (a)
2. Therapist passively flexes the knee (b)
   - Heel should almost touch or touch the buttock without any compensation (c)
   - PSIS pushes into the thumb
     - *Anterior tilt on the ipsilateral side*
     - *Tight rectus femoris*
   - Hip rotates
     - *Tight rectus femoris*
   - Hip abducts
     - *Tight rectus femoris*
   - Therapist needs to address any length deficiencies in rectus femoris
3. Address rectus femoris length
4. Pain in the lumbar spine? May be due to:
   - Femoral nerve irritation due to lumbosacral lesion or hip lesion
   - Potential protruding or bulging disc
   - Potential SIJ dysfunction
   - Athlete must be very specific with regard to location of pain
5. Refer patient to relevant practitioner if this is beyond your scope of practice.

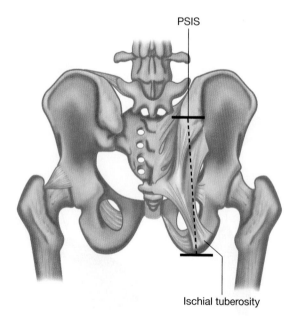

Figure 5.9: Position of the PSIS

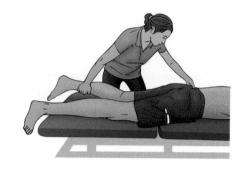

(a)

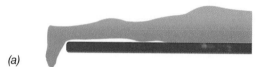

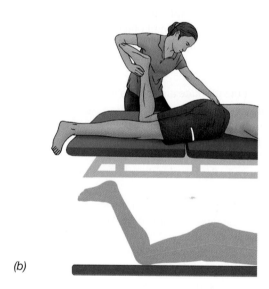

(b)

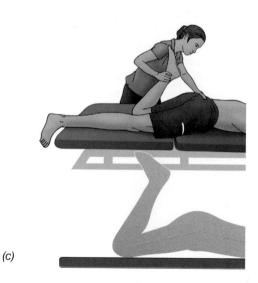

(c)

Figure 5.10: Position of therapist's finger and thumb on the PSIS for Ely's test

Assessment

In the last decade, clinical assessment procedures for the pelvic girdle have altered from simply testing the functional mobility of the SIJ to functional assessment procedures that test the ability of the pelvis to maintain stability during load transfer between the spine and the lower extremity (Hungerford et al., 2007). One of the reasons these tests have evolved is the increased knowledge of how the pelvis reacts to load transfer, and another relates to the poor reliability and validity of many SIJ mobility tests.

A systematic review and meta-analysis showed that there is discriminative power for diagnosing SIJ pain in the thigh-thrust test, in the compression test, and in three or more positive stress tests (see page 62). Because a gold standard for SIJ pain diagnosis is lacking, the diagnostic validity of tests related to the International Association for the Study of Pain criteria for SIJ pain should be regarded with care (Szadek et al., 2009). Recent evidence suggests that a cluster of tests for SIJ pain or dysfunction is necessary (Laslett et al., 2005; Robinson et al., 2007).

Mangen and Folia's (2009) systematic review suggests that because the thigh-thrust and distraction tests have the highest individual sensitivity and specificity, respectively, performance of these tests first seems reasonable. They indicate that should both tests elicit familiar pain, no further testing is indicated.

Mangen and Folia (2009) also suggest that should compression not be painful the sacral-thrust test should be applied. If this test proves to be painful, SIJ pathology is likely. If the sacral-thrust test is not painful, SIJ involvement is unlikely. The benefit of this is that addressing the SIJ in this way avoids having to subject patients/athletes/clients to unnecessary tests and, in the majority of cases, allows for a diagnosis even if one or more tests were not completed.

With limited movement in the SIJ it is of paramount importance to include a thorough evaluation of the lumbar spine, the hips (above and below joints), and the neurodynamic system before definitively deciding that the SIJ is the likely cause of the symptoms being presented (Sturesson et al., 2000).

The pelvic girdle receives its stability from the interconnection between the symphysis pubis and the SIJ, a strong ligamentous system, and the wedge shape of the sacrum, fitting vertically between the innominates (Hengevald and Banks, 2014). These structures produce a self-locking system (Kapandji, 2007) contributing to the form closure of the pelvis. Also contributing to the dynamic stability and therefore dynamic force closure of the pelvic girdle are a number of muscles groups and fascia.

Vleeming (1997) describes form closure as "the stable situation due to closely fitting joint surfaces, where no additional forces are necessary in order to maintain that state once it is under certain load." This is due to the shape and form of the sacrum, which is wedged between the two ilia.

The transversus abdominis (TA) contributes to pelvic stiffness owing to its anatomical attachments (to the innominate, and to the middle layer and deep lamina of the posterior layer of the thoracolumbar fascia (TLF)). The synergy of pelvic floor muscle contraction and co-contraction of the TA and multifidi increases stiffness, reduces shear forces in the SIJ, and contributes to stabilization of the pelvis, allowing correct load transfer in the lumbopelvic region to be maintained (Pel et al., 2008).

Musculature Slings

Lee (2004) describes four slings of global muscle groups that stabilize the pelvis regionally:

- The lateral sling
- The posterior oblique sling
- The anterior oblique sling
- The posterior longitudinal sling

The above slings by no means function in isolation; they interconnect, partially overlap, and function together (Lee, 2004). These slings may not influence spinal movement like the local stabilizing system does, but they can generate tension in the TLF adding to posterior pelvic compression and the control of rotation and shear within the lumbopelvic region.

There are multiple slings of muscles that envelop the SIJ, allowing it to be stabilized. The anatomical pattern of these slings gives the premise that rehabilitation can be performed on these muscles in an attempt to create SIJ stability. If a rehabilitation program is created to strengthen these muscles, the movement and pain from the SIJ may be reduced.

The 'slings' providing force closure in the pelvis include the posterior oblique sling, the anterior oblique sling and the posterior longitudinal sling, made up of the following structures:

Three Musculature Slings

The *posterior longitudinal sling* (see Figure 5.11) includes: multifidus (MF), the sacrum, the deep layer of the thoracolumbar fascia (TLF), the sacrotuberous ligament (STL), and biceps femoris (Hengevald and Banks, 2014).

- Erector spinae and MF are part of the deep longitudinal sling that simultaneously contribute to compression of the lumbar segments and provide a dynamic restraint to anterior/posterior shear stresses in the lumbar spine.
- The muscles making up this sling increase tension in the TLF and compress the SIJ.
- Biceps femoris can influence sacral nutation through its connection to the STL and plays a role in the intrinsic and extrinsic stability of the pelvis in relation to the leg (Vleeming et al., 2008).

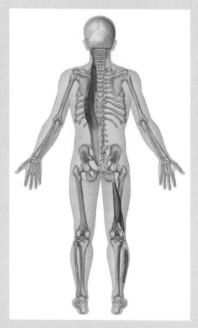

Figure 5.11: The posterior longitudinal sling

The *posterior oblique sling* (see Figure 5.12) has been shown to affect force closure, and includes latissimus dorsi, the TLF, and gluteus maximus (GM). The relationship between the posterior oblique sling and the SIJ is as follows:

- GM has the greatest capacity for force closure via the posterior layer of the TLF, and has been noted to transmit tension directly behind the SIJ as low as the third sacral vertebra (S3) (Barker et al., 2004).
- Van Wingerden et al. (2004) report that GM contraction increases stiffness at the SIJ threefold when combined with the contraction of latissimus dorsi during gait.

- Rotation against resistance has been found to activate the posterior oblique sling (Vleeming and Stoeckart, 2007).
- GM creates a muscle link between the tensor fascia lata and the TLF. Contraction of the GM increases stiffness in the fascia that spans the lumbar spine, SIJ, and hips (Hengevald and Banks, 2014).
- Hungerford et al. (2003) have found that the onset of contraction of GM is altered with SIJ dysfunction.

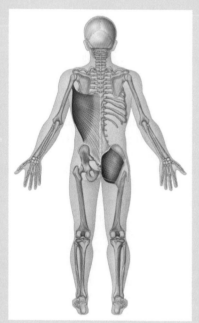

Figure 5.12: The posterior oblique sling

The *anterior oblique sling* (see Figure 5.13) includes the external obliques, internal obliques, transversus abdominis, rectus abdominis, linea alba, inguinal ligament, and the adductors.

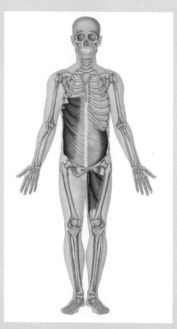

Figure 5.13: The anterior oblique sling

Further Considerations Before Commencing Treatment

The fascial lines (Myers, 2001) also need to be taken into consideration when looking at dysfunction and function around the pelvis. The erector spinae muscles, along with multifidus, simultaneously contribute to compression of the lumbar segments and provide a dynamic restraint to anterior–posterior shear stresses in the lumbar spine (Myers, 2001). The muscles in this sling increase tension throughout the TLF and compress the SIJ. Biceps femoris can influence sacral nutation through its connection to the sacrotuberous ligament.

Hypertonic global muscles can contribute to dysfunctional adaptation strategies around the pelvis. Chest gripping indicates hyperactivity in the obliques, back gripping indicates hyperactivity in the erector spinae, and bottom gripping indicates hyperactivity in the piriformis and obturator internus. The strategies above are commonly witnessed in people who no longer have spinal, intrapelvic, and/or hip motion control (Lee, 2004). We need to be addressing these hypertonic tissues with soft-tissue work before we even think about rehabilitating the local muscles.

Without full ROM available at the lumbar spine and the hips, there may be excessive strain and compensation in the SIJ. Clearing the hips with a squat (first with the heels off the ground then with the heels on the ground) will assess full hip flexion in weight bearing. Concentrate on how much flexion is produced in the lumbar spine (increased lumbar flexion can be indicative of hip flexion restriction). In addition, test for how much range is available in hip flexion and extension by asking your patient to lunge with one foot on the edge of a chair or low plinth and observing any compensation strategies present in the spine or innominates.

Commonly, the complaints from people struggling with an SIJ disorder include pain and heaviness or fatigue in the leg on the affected side, particularly during weight-bearing activities. The pain is described as being sudden and sharp preventing some people from going about their activities of daily living (ADL).

SIJ symptoms rarely travel over to the contralateral side; these are usually isolated to the posterior aspect of the SIJ in question and can refer as far down as the calf and foot, but often refer into to the buttocks, the groin, and around the posterior thigh.

SIJ pain often has people adapting their position to reduce the symptoms they are experiencing; these can include regularly having to lean to the side and sit on one buttock or sitting with the legs crossed. You may witness when assessing sit to stand (STS) that your patient has to push the knees together for support in order to stand, in addition to pushing on the pelvis. It is also not uncommon for people with dysfunctional SIJs to want to sink their knuckles into their lower back, glute, or sacral/SIJ area to attempt to alleviate the discomfort they are experiencing. All of these are clues, and help you with your clinical reasoning hypothesis.

Potential Activity Restrictions due to SIJ Pain

Mens et al. (2001) looked at activity restriction due to pain arising from the SIJ. By knowing these functional activities you can tailor the subjective questioning to delve deeper into the history of the patient's present condition:

- Ninety percent of patients described pain when standing for thirty minutes (static loading).
- Eighty-six percent of patients described pain when carrying a full shopping bag (dynamic loading).
- Eighty-one percent of patients described pain when single-leg standing (shear forces with load).
- Eighty-one percent of patients described pain when walking for thirty minutes (dynamic loading and shear forces).

Assessing the Pelvis

Positional analysis of the pelvic girdle should be made prior to assessing joint mobility, as differences in mobility may just be a reflection of a different bony starting position. The pelvis is subjected to multiple force vectors from the muscles that attach to it and these can impact on its position.

It is also important to take into consideration that the primary function of the lumbopelvic-hip complex is to transfer loads safely while fulfilling the movement and control requirements of a task.

Lee and Lee (2010) suggest the following for effective palpation of the ilia, sacrum, and ischia. Assessments should be done in supine and prone positions, using the entire hand (to more accurately assess the position).

Palpation of the Iliac Crests

Supine:
- Legs extended
- Place heels of hands on lateral aspect of innominates
- Note any differences
- Position can be confirmed by placing thumbs on the inferior aspect of the anterior superior iliac spine (ASIS).

Prone:
- Legs extended
- Palpate both innominates with the heels of the hands on the inferior aspect of the posterior superior iliac spine (PSIS) and the rest of the hand on the back of the innominates
- Can you detect any differences in the positions when comparing left to right?
- Position can be confirmed by placing the thumbs on the inferior aspect of the PSIS.

Ischial tuberosities can also be used to confirm any vertical shear of one innominate relative to the other. The most inferior aspect of the ischial tuberosities is palpated bilaterally with the thumbs.

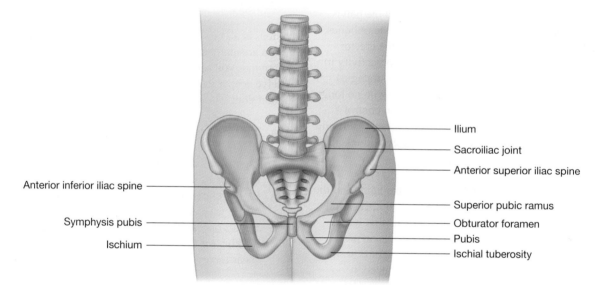

Figure 5.14: Landmarks of the pelvis, anterior view

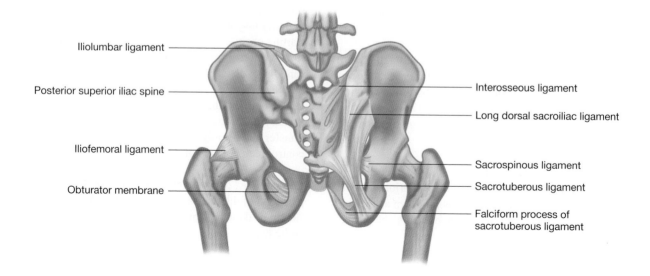

Figure 5.15: Ligaments of the pelvis, posterior view

Palpation of the SIJ

- The SIJ is located between the sacrum and the ilium (deep to the thoracolumbar fascia)
- It is medial to the PSIS
- Palpate in prone—locate the PSIS
- Travel inferomedially to locate the joint
- Flex the ipsilateral knee and take hold of the foot
- Rotate the hip medially and laterally
- Feel for the small opening in the joint space.

The pelvic girdle functions synergistically with the lumbar spine and the hips, and the SIJ needs perfect balance between movement and stability (see Figure 5.16). The structures surrounding the joint (muscles, fascia, ligaments) provide "force closure," allowing both movement and stability.

Descending forces

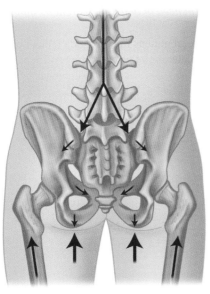

Ascending forces

Figure 5.16: The SIJ needs perfect balance between movement and stability

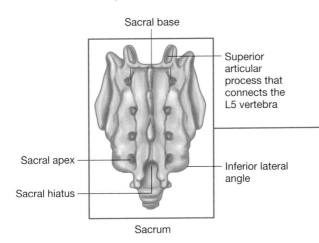

Sacral base

Superior articular process that connects the L5 vertebra

Sacral apex

Inferior lateral angle

Sacral hiatus

Sacrum

Position of Sacrum

- Prone, legs extended
- Palpate dorsal aspect of the inferior lateral angles of the sacrum
- Assess any rotation
- Lee and Lee (2010) state that this bony point appears more reliable for assessing the position of the sacrum as the sacral base depth can be influenced by the size and tone of the sacral multifidus.

Commonly, the people who come seeking treatment struggle to recruit the local muscles (deep, segmental, stabilizers) owing to the dominance and overactivity of the global muscles (cross over many segments or regions, movers and general stabilizers). Therefore, we need to tackle the global muscle dysfunction first; this is often what is causing the inhibition of the local muscles.

The main group of local muscles that generates tension to stabilize the lumbar spine and pelvic girdle includes transversus abdominis, the deep fibers of multifidus, the pelvic floor, the diaphragm, and the posterior fibers of the psoas major (Gibbons, 2001). When dysfunction is present in these structures there will be delays in the timing of contraction, visible or palpable atrophy (loss of tone), or loss of coordination when attempting to work alongside other local muscles. When dysfunction is present in the structures of the global muscle system there will be evidence of dominance, co-contraction, hypertonicity, delayed activation, weakness, poor recruitment, loss of synergy when moving, and a reduction in flexibility.

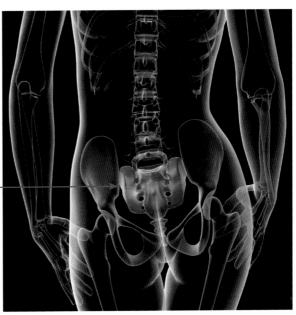

Figure 5.17: Position of the sacrum

SIJ Anatomy

- The SIJ is a synovial (anterior) and fibrous (posterior) joint between the articular surface of the ilium and the ala of the sacrum.
- A fibrous capsule completely surrounds the joint, investing into the tissues on the articular margins of both bones.
- The joint is richly endowed with ligaments (surrounding the capsule), which are extremely strong posteriorly and slightly weaker anteriorly.
- Accessory ligaments provide additional stability (sacrotuberous, sacrospinous, iliolumbar)

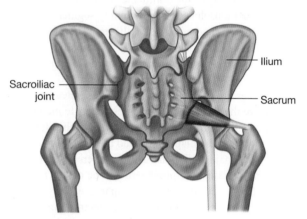

Figure 5.18: The sacroiliac joint

Self-Locking Ability of the SIJ

When the sacrum rests on the dorsal sacral ligaments during nutation, tension and stability are created for the SIJ. However, when the sacrotuberous ligament (STL) is loaded (e.g. tension in biceps femoris, GM, piriformis, and TLF), SIJ mobility is decreased. Interestingly, a connection can be made between pregnant women and tight hamstrings—the hamstrings attempt to load the STL, working harder to keep the now-mobile SIJ stable (Kapandji, 2007).

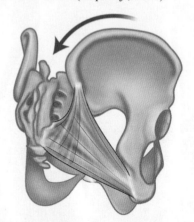

Figure 5.19: Sacrotuberous ligament tensioned, limiting SIJ mobility

Joint Ranges of Motion Common with SIJ Dysfunction

- Reduced knee extension
- Reduced hip internal rotation
- Reduced hip external rotation
- Reduced hip extension
- Reduced hip flexion

Soft-Tissue Findings Common with SIJ Dysfunction

Hypertonic (in need of soft-tissue input):

- Ipsilateral piriformis, biceps femoris, adductor magnus, quadratus lumborum and obliques
- Contralateral iliacus, latissimus dorsi and adductors

Inhibited (in need of activation/strengthening):

- Ipsilateral gluteus medius and erector spinae
- Contralateral gluteus maximus and psoas major

Assessing for Pain

The latest research strongly supports pain provocation tests as these have shown good reliability individually, but even more so when two or three are done together (Laslett and Williams, 1994, 2005; van der Wurff et al., 2000a, b; Robinson et al., 2007).

The most relevant and most recent evidence shows that a minimum of three SIJ pain-provocation tests must reproduce the patient's pain before the pain can be considered as originating from the SIJ (Szadek et al., 2009).

- Distraction test
- Compression test
- Thigh-thrust test
- Sacral-thrust test.

Distraction Test

(This is the most specific test (Laslett et al., 2005).)

1. Athlete supine, lying with small pillow under knees (to keep the lumbar spine in neutral)
2. Heels of hands on medial aspects of both ASIS Perform a slow steady posterolateral force through both ASIS (distracting the anterior part of the SIJ and compressing the posterior part)
3. Maintain this force
4. Ask athlete about reproduction and localization of pain.

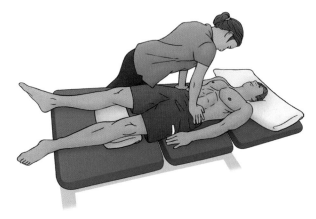

Figure 5.20: Distraction test

Compression Test

1. Side-lying position, hips and knees flexed
2. Place both hands over the anterolateral iliac crest
3. Apply a slow steady medial force through the innominate—compressing the anterior part of the SIJ and distracting the posterior part
4. Maintain force
5. Ask patient about reproduction of pain
6. Repeat test both sides.

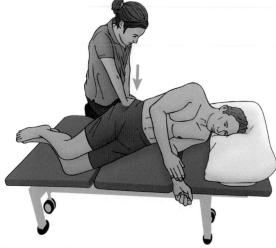

Figure 5.21: Compression test

Thigh-Thrust Test

Attempting to elicit pain whilst performing a posterior shearing force to the SIJ of that side.

1. Athlete supine with the hip and knee flexed
2. Thigh ninety degrees to the plinth and slightly adducted
3. Therapist's hand cups the sacrum, the other arm and hand wrap around the flexed knee
4. Therapist applies pressure down toward the plinth along the line of the vertically oriented femur
5. Repeat both sides.

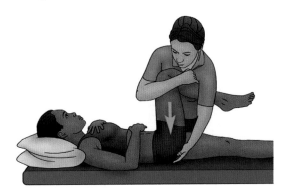

Figure 5.22: Thigh-thrust test

Sacral-Thrust Test

Attempting to elicit pain whilst performing an anterior shearing force of the sacrum on both ilia.

1. Athlete in prone position
2. Therapist applies a force vertically downward to the center of the sacrum.

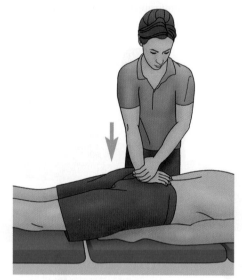

Figure 5.23: Sacral-thrust test

Additional Test

Gaenslen's Test

1. Athlete supine near the edge of the couch
2. Patient's hip is fully flexed into the abdomen and held there by the patient as the therapist adds overpressure
3. The opposite leg is slowly hyperextended by the therapist over the edge of the bed with overpressure over the knee
4. Test is positive when pain is reproduced over the flexed side.

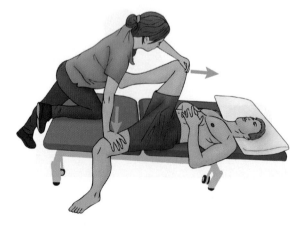

Figure 5.24: Gaenslen's test

Assessing for Loss of Function

Stork Test

The stork test (aka modified Trendelenberg/one-leg standing (OLS)/Gillet) and the active straight-leg raise test (ASLR) have both shown acceptable inter-tester reliability. Lee and Lee (2010) also assess lateral tilts of the pelvis in both supine and standing positions to test load transfer through the symphysis pubis.

The stork test (see Figure 5.25) is a motion-control test where both form and force closure mechanisms are assessed by observing how load is managed through the pelvis in standing. The ability to maintain a stable alignment of the ilium relative to the sacrum when testing the weight-bearing side (self-braced alignment of the pelvic bones) is what is expected. There should be no relative movement occurring in the pelvis during this load-transfer test (this test is also utilized as a symphysis pubis pain-provocation test) and it should be performed three times to ensure that the same pattern is observed.

The ability of the non-weight-bearing side (NWB) innominate to rotate posteriorly relative to the ipsilateral sacrum can also be assessed by this test (Hungerford et al., 2007; Lee and Lee, 2010). Observe the quality of the symmetry between both sides.
How to perform:

1. Athlete standing
2. Kneel behind the athlete, and place the heel of your hand on the ilium of the side to be tested
3. Wrap the fingers of that same hand around the ilium and keep them relaxed
   - Place the thumb of the same hand just below the posterior superior iliac spine (PSIS)
   - Place the contralateral (other hand) thumb at S2
   - Keep both hands relaxed
4. Ask the patient to stand on one leg (the side you are assessing) and bring their knee in line with the belly button
5. Repeat three times—are you getting the same results each time?
6. Repeat on the other side (remembering to change your hands around) as you always need a comparison
7. Is the effort the same on both sides?
8. Was the transfer of weight onto the weight-bearing (WB) leg smooth?
9. Did the pelvis stay in the same position?
10. This can also be done leaving the hands in the same position, but placed this time on the side of the body where the hip is being flexed (NWB side)

11. The thumb placed below the PSIS should drop below its original position as the pelvis is rotated backward relative to the sacrum during hip flexion
12. Again compare to the contralateral side, looking for symmetry.

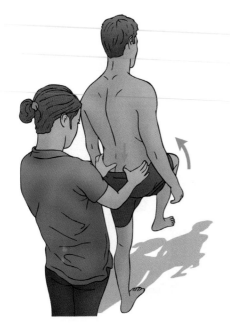

Figure 5.25: The stork test

Active Straight-Leg Raise (ASLR)

Assesses load through the pelvis in supine position.

1. Athlete lifts the nonaffected leg eight inches from the bed and compares the difference in effort experienced when lifting the leg of the affected side
2. The effort can be scored on a scale of 0–5 (Mens et al., 2001)
3. The leg should feel light when lifting it off the plinth; there should be no movement of the pelvis in any direction in relation to the trunk or the legs
4. If this is too difficult or the leg feels heavy, this indicates poor recruitment of both local and global muscles.

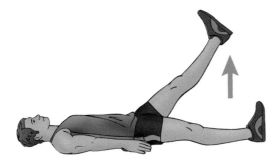

Figure 5.26: Active straight-leg raise (ASLR)

The Role of the Psoas in the ASLR

Hu et al. (2011) investigated the role of the psoas in hip flexion using the ASLR test (hip flexion pulls the innominate forward). Historically, this action was considered as being counteracted by the contralateral biceps femoris and the ipsilateral lateral abdominals (pressing the innominate toward the sacrum for increased force closure). Their results highlighted that problems with the ASLR may reflect problems with force closure, abdominal wall activation counterbalances forward rotation of the innominate, and contralateral biceps femoris activation leads to transverse plane rotation of the pelvis (clinically seen as an upward movement of the contralateral ASIS). This, in turn, is counteracted by the ipsilateral transversus abdominis and internal oblique; the psoas is active bilaterally (potentially reflecting its stabilizing of the lumbar spine); iliacus, rectus femoris, and adductor longus are active ipsilaterally (synergistically).

The addition of compression to the pelvis (squeezing of the anterior portion of the innominates, or bringing the ASIS closer together) can enable the leg to be lifted with ease (unless there is already too much compression, in which case this movement may be made even more difficult).

Altering the location of the compression forces can assist the therapist in determining where more compression is needed (and where weakness is present) functionally to help load transfer through the pelvic girdle (Lee and Lee, 2010) and therefore plan an effective treatment program.

Lee and Lee (2010) suggest compression differences in different areas of the pelvis:

- Anterior compression—squeezing the ASIS closer together (stimulates transversus abdominis (TA))
- Anterior compression above the greater trochanter of the hips (stimulates anterior pelvic floor)
- Posterior compression—bringing both PSIS together (stimulates multifidus)
- Anterior compression of left ASIS and posterior compression of right PSIS toward each other (stimulates left TA and right multifidus).

The compression that is noted to be most helpful for the patient during the ASLR test should be kept in mind when planning the treatment.

Keep in mind that if there is too much compression the patient will not do well or may find the task of lifting the leg even more difficult.

What if you find that compression (force closure) is reduced?

1. Assess and treat lumbar spine and hips, as these are likely to be hypomobile
   - Compensation or strain on the structures impacting on the SIJ
2. Temporary use of an SIJ belt
3. Walking and swimming activates gluteus maximus
   - Increases tension on the thoracolumbar fascia (TLF)
4. Specific training of gluteus maximus and latissimus dorsi (posterior oblique sling), erector spinae and multifidus (Vleeming and Stoeckart, 2007)
   - Assists force closure
   - Strengthens TLF.

What if you find that compression (force closure) in excessive?

1. Overactive global muscles in the lumbopelvic region compressing SIJ?
2. Pain-provocation tests positive?
3. Stork test negative?
4. ASLR negative?
5. Assess and treat connective tissue around the SIJ
   - Soft-tissue work (connective tissue)
   - Hip external rotators if bottom gripping is apparent
   - Muscle energy techniques (MET)
   - Mobilizations and mobility exercises
   - Postural training
6. Reduce hypertonicity in dominant global muscles
7. Stop stabilization exercises (muscles are already too active)
8. Add in breathing exercises:
   - Costolateral, diaphragmatic breathing.

Additional SIJ Function Tests

(These tests have reduced sensitivity and specificity.)

Standing Flexion Test

1. Athlete standing
2. Stand behind the athlete, and:
   - Place the heels of both hands on the ilia
   - Wrap the fingers around the ilia and keep them relaxed
   - Place the thumbs just below the PSIS
   - Keep both hands relaxed
3. Ask the patient to bend forward as far as they can go (see Figure 5.27)
4. Repeat three times—are you getting the same results each time?
5. Compare sides, looking for symmetry

- If the thumbs stay level (move equal distance) during flexion, this is normal/negative
- If the PSIS moves in cephalad direction on one side during flexion this is indicative of SIJ dysfunction/limited movement of the sacrum on the ilium on that side.

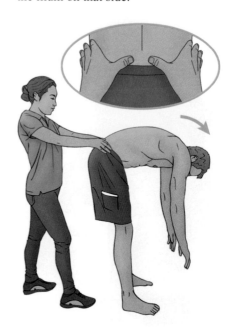

Figure 5.27: Standing flexion test

Seated Flexion Test

1. Athlete seated in the middle of the plinth with feet touching the floor
2. Kneel behind athlete, and:
   - Place the heels of both hands on the ilia
   - Wrap the fingers around the ilia and keep them relaxed
   - Place the thumbs just below the PSIS
   - Keep both hands relaxed
3. Ask the patient to bend forward as far as they can go (see Figure 5.28)
4. Repeat three times—are you getting the same results each time?
5. Compare sides, looking for symmetry
   - If the thumbs stay level (move equal distance) during flexion, this is normal/negative
   - If the PSIS moves in cephalad direction on one side during flexion this is indicative of SIJ dysfunction/limited movement of the sacrum on the ilium on that side.

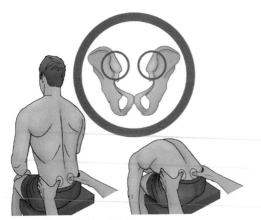

Figure 5.28: Seated flexion test

Hip-Abduction Test

1. Indicated in screening for stability of lumbopelvic region
2. Athlete side-lying with lower hip and knee flexed and upper leg extended
3. Leg is lifted actively into abduction
4. Leg should abduct approximately twenty degrees
5. There should be no external rotation (ER), hip flexion, or hip hitching
6. Moderate lumbar erector spinae/quadratus lumborum (QL) contraction is allowed
7. Positive result if:
   - ER in femur is present—shortening of piriformis
   - ER of pelvis—piriformis and other lateral rotator overactivity/shortness
   - Hip flexion occurs—psoas, tensor fascia latae (TFL) overactivity/shortness
   - Hitching of pelvis before twenty degrees of hip abduction—QL overactivity/shortening
   - Pain in ipsilateral adductor—adductors shortened.

Hip-Extension Test

1. Indicated in assessing coordinated muscle activation during prone hip extension
2. Athlete prone with arms relaxed
3. Feet extended beyond plinth
4. Leg is lifted into extension
5. Initial contraction is expected in the thoracolumbar erector spinae muscles (stabilizing torso)
6. Full action should be achieved by coordinated activity of the hamstrings and gluteus maximus (GM)
7. Positive result if:
   - Knee flexes—indicative of hamstring shortness
   - Delayed/absent (inhibited) GM firing—indicative of overactivity of erector spinae muscles +/– hamstring muscles
   - False hip extension—lower back performs this movement—indicative of inhibited GM or erector spinae overactivity
   - Premature contralateral periscapular muscular contraction—indicative of functional lower back instability (recruiting upper torso to compensate for prime mover inhibition).

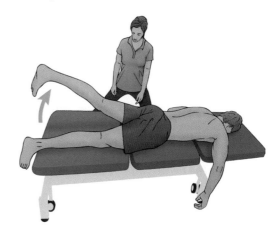

Figure 5.30: Hip-extension test

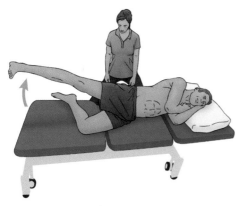

Figure 5.29: Hip-abduction test

References

Gibbons SCT, Pelley B, and Molgaard J (2001) Biomechanics and stability mechanisms of psoas major. *Proceedings of 4th Interdisciplinary World Conference on Low Back Pain*, Montreal, Canada, November 9–11, 2001

Hengeveld E and Banks K (2014) *Maitland's Peripheral Manipulation*. Oxford, Churchill Livingstone

Hu H, Meijer OG, van Dieën JH, Hodges PW, Bruijn SM, Strijers RL, and Xia C (2011) Is the psoas a hip flexor in the active straight leg raise? *European Spine Journal* 20(5): 759–765

Hungerford B, Gilleard W, and Hodges P (2003) Evidence of altered lumbopelvic muscle recruitment in the presence of sacroiliac joint pain. *Spine* 28: 1593–1600

Hungerford B, Gilleard W, and Moran M (2007) Evaluation of the ability of physical therapists to palpate intrapelvic motion with the stork test on the support side. *Physical Therapy* 87(7): 879–887

Janda V (1992) Treatment of chronic back pain. *Journal of Manual Medicine* 6: 166–168

Kapandji I (2007) *The Physiology of the Joints*. Edinburgh, Churchill Livingstone

Laslett M, Aprill CN, McDonald B, and Young SB (2005) Diagnosis of sacroilial joint pain: validity of individual provocation tests and composites of tests. *Manual Therapy* 10: 207–218

Laslett M, van der Wurff P, Buijs EJ, Aprill C (2007) Comments on Berthelot et al. review: "Provocative sacroiliac joint maneuvers and sacroiliac joint block are unreliable for diagnosing sacroiliac joint pain." *Joint, Bone Spine* 74: 306–307

Lee D (2004) *The Pelvic Girdle*. Edinburgh, Churchill Livingstone

Lee D and Lee L (2010). *The Pelvic Girdle*. Edinburgh, Elsevier/Churchill Livingstone

Majlesi J, Togay H, Ünalan H, and Tprak S (2008) The sensitivity and specificity of the slump and the straight leg raising tests in patients with lumbar disc herniation. *Journal of Clinical Rheumatology* 14(2): 87–91

Mangen J and Folia V (2009) Validity of clinical tests for sacroiliac and lumbar joint dysfunction: a systematic review of the literature. *Systematic Reviews* 1: 1–35

Mens JM, Vleeming A, Snijders CJ, Koes BW, and Stam HJ (2001) Reliability and validity of the active straight leg raise test in posterior pelvic pain since pregnancy. *Spine* 26(10): 1167–1171

Myers T (2001) *Anatomy Trains*. Edinburgh, Churchill Livingstone

Pel J, Spoor C, Pool-Goudzwaard A, Hoek van Dijke G, and Snijders C (2008) Biomechanical analysis of reducing sacroiliac joint shear load by optimization of pelvic muscle and ligament forces. *Annals of Biomedical Engineering* 36(3): 415–424

Robinson HS, Brox JI, Robinson R, Bjelland E, Solem S, and Telje T (2007) Technical and measurement report the reliability of selected motion- and pain-provocation tests for the sacroiliac joint. *Manual Therapy* 12: 72–79

Sturesson B, Uden A, and Vleeming A (2000) A radiostereometric analysis of movements of the sacroiliac joints during the standing hip flexion test. *Spine* 25: 364–368

Szadek K, van der Wurff P, van Tulder M, Zuurmond W, and Perez R (2009) Diagnostic validity of criteria for sacroiliac joint pain: a systematic review. *Journal of Pain* 10(4): 354–368

van der Wurff O, Hagmeijer RHM, and Meyne W (2000a) Clinical tests of the sacroiliac joint: a systematic methodological review—Part 1: Reliability. *Manual Therapy* 5(1): 30–36

van der Wurff O, Hagmeijer RHM, and Meyne W (2000b) Clinical tests of the sacroiliac joint: a systematic methodological review—Part 2: Validity. *Manual Therapy* 5(2): 89–96

van Wingerden JP, Vleeming A, Buyruk HM, and Raissadat K (2004) Stabilization of the SIJ in vivo: verification of muscular contribution to force closure of the pelvis. *European Spine Journal* 13(3): 199

Vleeming A and Stoeckart R (2007) The role of the pelvic girdle in coupling the spine and the legs: a clinical-anatomical perspective on pelvic stability. In: Vleeming A, Mooney V, and Stoeckart R (eds) *Movement, Stability and Lumbopelvic Pain: Integration and Research*. Edinburgh, Churchill Livingstone.

Posterior Oblique Sling

Latissimus Dorsi

Attachments

- Posterior layer of the thoracolumbar fascia invests into the spinous processes of the lower six thoracic and all of the lumbar and sacral vertebrae, and to the supraspinatus and interspinous ligaments
- Arises from the fascia of the posterior part of the outer lip of the iliac crest, sweeps upward and laterally across the lower part of the thorax, then invests into the periosteum surrounding the lower three of four ribs and via fascia to the inferior angle of the scapula
- The fibers then converge as they pass to the humerus and form a thin flattened tendon
- The tendon winds around and adheres to the lower border of teres major and invests into the floor of the intertubercular groove, anterior to the tendon of teres major (separated by a bursa)
- The effect of twisting the muscle through one hundred and eighty degrees means that the anterior surface of the tendon is continuous with the posterior surface of the rest of the muscle
- The fibers with the lowest attachments on the trunk gain the highest attachment on the humeral periosteum.

Innervation

- Thoracodorsal nerve (root value C6–8)
- Skin covering the muscle (roots T4–12, L1–3).

Action

- Strong extensor of the flexed arm
- If humerus is fixed relative to the scapula, latissimus dorsi retracts the pectoral girdle
- Strong adductor and medial rotator of the humerus at the shoulder joint
- With arms fixed above the head, latissimus dorsi can raise the trunk upward (with pectoralis major)
- Used in rowing and the downstroke in swimming
- Owing to the relationship with the ribs, latissimus dorsi is active in violent expiration (cough or sneeze)
- If the humerus is fixed, when using crutches for example, latissimus dorsi is able to pull the trunk forward relative to the arms (attaches via fascia to the pelvis).

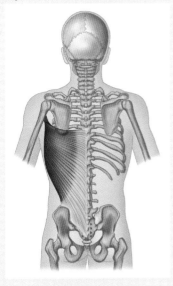

Figure 6.1: Latissimus dorsi

Therapy Input

When performing all of the soft-tissue inputs below, please take into consideration the points highlighted in Chapter 2: Fascia, regarding the speed at which to move deeper into the tissues. I use a maximum VAS[1] score of 6/10 (athlete's perception) when sinking into tissues, so as not to elicit a resistant tissue response and so as not to cause "pain" to the athlete. My perception of 6/10 is a moderate discomfort (which does not elicit escaping maneuvers by the athlete, pulling away); I explain to the athlete that there is no need to be "brave" and that there will be no sudden movements or increase in pressure once I have reached this depth. Achieving the depth is a gradual process, controlled by the athlete and by the tissue response, and it can take more than sixty seconds before tissue response is felt or the athlete feels a reduction in discomfort. At this point I advise the athlete to let me know when the discomfort has "dropped" to approximately 2/10.

Following this, I add the active or passive movement of a body part. I advise the athlete that a movement causing discomfort above 6/10 will be stopped at that location, until the discomfort drops to 2/10 and completion of the movement may commence. I then repeat this until all the relevant tissues have been addressed.

I have not repeated these statements in the directions below, but please accept that they are to be repeated any time you are working deeply into the tissues.

Palpation

1. Athlete prone.
2. Arms at ninety degrees of abduction.
3. Grasp the tissue between the lateral border of the scapula and the abducted humerus.
4. Athlete medially rotates the shoulder as you resist (to confirm location).
5. Palpate over the ribs and into the axilla.

Assessment for Length (see figure 6.2)

1. Athlete standing or supine with hips and knees flexed.
2. If the athlete is unable to fully flex the shoulder, and there is no underlying shoulder pathology, the movement is stopped and the range is noted.
3. Athlete flexes both upper limbs in the sagittal plane.
   - If the lower back arches, the movement is stopped and the range is noted
   - If the athlete is unable to fully flex the shoulder, the movement is stopped and the range is noted
   - Indicative of short latissimus dorsi.
4. Worthy of note:
   - Pectoralis minor may place scapula in anterior tilt producing the same result
   - Anterior abdominals may be tight, therefore depressing the thorax and pulling scapula anteriorly.
5. Reassess after treatment.

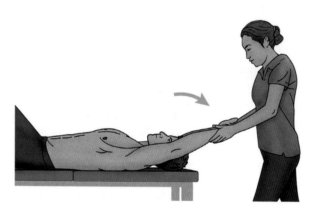

Figure 6.2: Assessment of latissimus dorsi for length

Assessment for Strength

1. Athlete prone.
2. Shoulder slightly abducted and elbow flexed.
3. Stabilize athlete's thorax.
4. Athlete extends the shoulder against your resistance.
5. Graded:
   - 5/5—strong contraction (normal)
   - 4/5—firm contraction (good)
   - 3/5—soft contraction (fair)
   - 2/5—slight contraction (poor)
   - 1/5—flicker (trace)
   - 0/5—no contraction detected.
6. Weakness may be due to inhibition, trigger points, pain, muscle length, neurological deficits.
7. Reassess after treatment.

---

1. VAS—visual analogue scale (see Glossary, Chapter 1).

Soft-Tissue Treatment: Athlete Prone

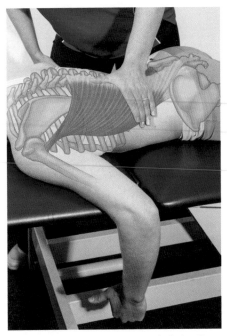

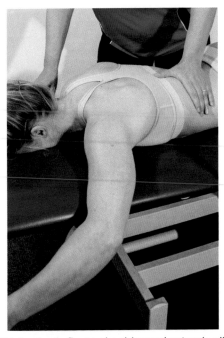

1. *With arm in forty-five degrees of abduction, elbow flexed, thumb in "thumbs up" position (this thumb position is maintained throughout to ensure external rotation of the shoulder).*
2. *Using a broad hand grip, slowly melt into the fascia (emerging from the posterior part of the outer lip of the iliac crest, which sweeps upward and laterally across the lower part of the thorax).*

3. *Athlete slowly flexes shoulder and extends elbow (arm taken in line with the ipsilateral ear).*
   - *Facilitate the movement by following with the contact hand (pressure maintained)—good for painful movements initially.*
   - *Resist the movement by locking into the tissues, maintaining that position whilst the tissues are actively or passively taken into position.*

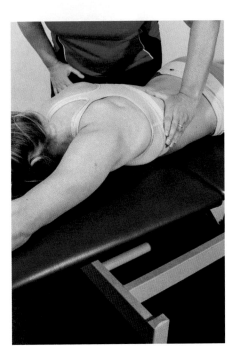

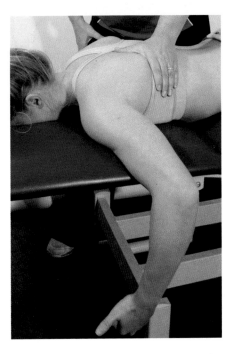

4. *Repeat until the palpable tissues of latissimus dorsi have been in contact with your hand.*

5. *Facilitation of the scapula movement at this stage is effective, following the exact principles above.*

Soft-Tissue Treatment: Athlete Side-Lying

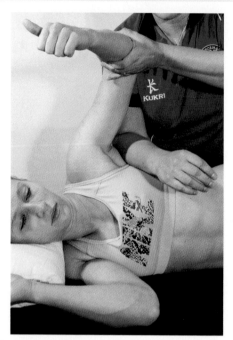

1. *Passively abduct the athlete's arm.*
2. *Using a broad hand grip or the ulnar border of the forearm, slowly melt into the tissues of the latissimus dorsi just before they merge into the humerus.*

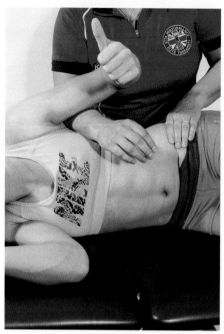

3. *The athlete's arm can now be returned (relaxed across the contact arm or hand).*

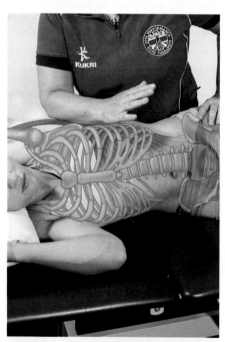

4. *Athlete slowly flexes the shoulder (thumb in "thumbs up" position—maintaining external rotation).*
   - *Facilitate the movement by following with the contact hand (pressure maintained)—good for painful movements initially.*
   - *Resist the movement by locking into the tissues, maintaining that position whilst the tissues are actively or passively taken into position.*

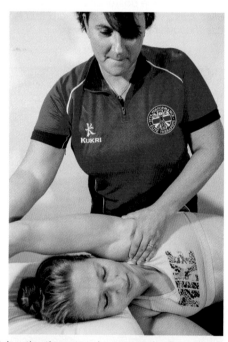

5. *Using the thenar eminence or the flat lateral surface of the thumb, reach up into the highest attachment of the latissimus dorsi and repeat the steps above.*

Soft-Tissue Treatment: Athlete Supine

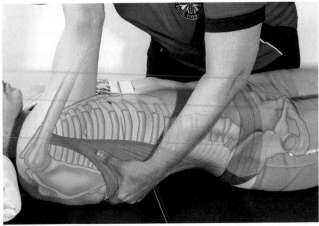

1. *Athlete flexes arm to ninety degrees.*
2. *With a broad thumb or palmar surface of the hand contact, slowly melt into the tissues of the latissimus dorsi where they merge into the humerus.*

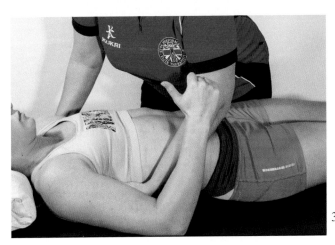

3. *Athlete returns the shoulder to approximately forty-five degrees of flexion.*

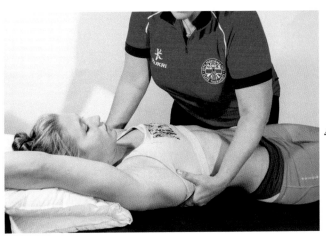

4. *Athlete slowly flexes and externally rotates the shoulder.*
   - *Facilitate the movement by following with the contact hand (pressure maintained)—good for painful movements initially.*
   - *Resist the movement by locking into the tissues, maintaining that position whilst the tissues are actively or passively taken into position.*

Dry Needling for Latissimus Dorsi

Dry needling should only be performed by a qualified and insured physical therapist owing to the invasive nature of the technique and serious anatomical considerations.

1. Athlete is prone/supine/side-lying.
2. Note referral pattern—does this represent your athletes pain?
3. Arm abducted to ninety degrees.
4. Grasp the tissues using a lumbrical grip (see Figure 6.4), lifting the tissues away from the ribs/chest wall.
5. Palpate the tissues for taut bands.
6. Insert the needle perpendicularly through the skin and into the taut band.

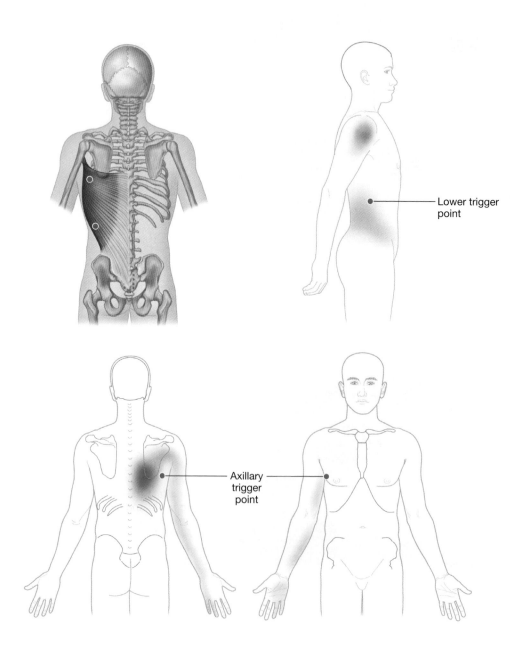

Figure 6.3: Latissimus dorsi trigger points and referral pattern

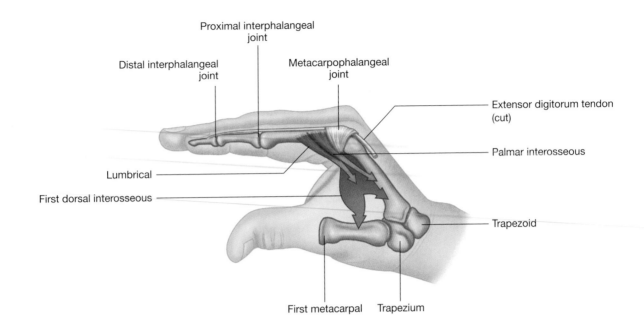

Figure 6.4: The combined action of the lumbricales and interossei is as flexors at the metacarpophalangeal (MCP) joint and extensors at the interphalangeal joints. The lumbricales have the greatest moment arm for flexion at the MCP joint

Instrument-Assisted Soft-Tissue Mobilization (IASTM)

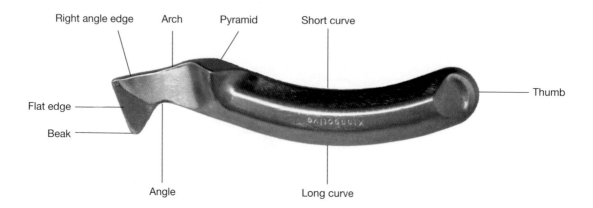

Figure 6.5: Instrument-assisted soft-tissue mobilization (IASTM) tool. The 3-D shape of the Kinnective tool has been developed with an emphasis for multifunctional treatments and the ability to provide flexible clinical applications. Only one instrument is required for all IASTM applications. The benefits of a single instrument are clear but usually necessitate a compromise on product; however, the Kinnective is specifically designed to produce optimal ergonomics, feedback, and flexible application in clinical practice

Instrument-Assisted Soft-Tissue Mobilization (IASTM): Athlete Side-Lying

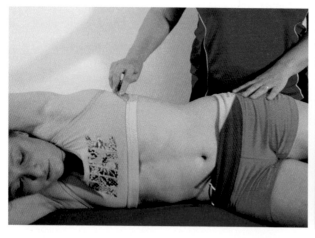 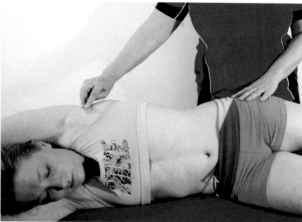

1. *Instrument to skin contact is necessary. Pictures are shown with clothing to protect the model's dignity.*
2. *Athlete positions ipsilateral upper and lower limb into extension.*
3. *Upper-arm extension gives easy access to the convergence of the upper fibers as they spiral into the axilla.*
4. *Take up the tissue slack and protect bony prominences and borders with the non-instrument hand.*
5. *Initially, scan the area using the long or short curve, identifying points of restriction or resistance.*
6. *Releasing tension between skin and superficial fascia:*
   - *Keep pressure light.*
   - *Keep strokes swift.*
7. *Athlete repeatedly extends arm and leg simultaneously during inspiration, relaxing on expiration.*
8. *When adding movement to re-establish sliding and gliding between layers, ensure the pressure is not pinning the tissues.*
9. *Using the thumb part of the instrument produces good specificity and accuracy.*

Instrument-Assisted Soft-Tissue Mobilization (IASTM): Athlete Seated

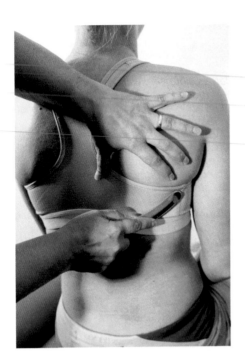

1. *Take up the tissue slack and protect bony prominences and borders with the non-instrument hand.*
2. *Initially, scan the area using the long or short curve, identifying points of restriction or resistance.*
3. *Releasing tension between skin and superficial fascia:*
   - *Keep pressure light.*
   - *Keep strokes swift.*

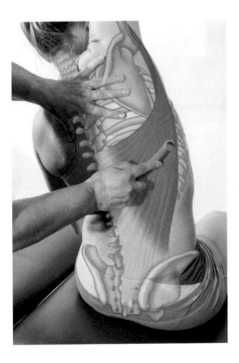

4. *Use broad strokes (using long curve) slowly sweeping upward and downward.*
   - *Instruct athlete to abduct the ipsilateral shoulder to one hundred and eighty degrees, simultaneously flexing the spine toward the contralateral side.*
5. *On your instruction, the athlete changes direction by simultaneously flexing the spine contralaterally and horizontally adducting the arm.*
6. *Repeat the broad sweeps, avoiding producing red bruising.*

Muscle Energy Techniques (MET): Athlete Side-Lying

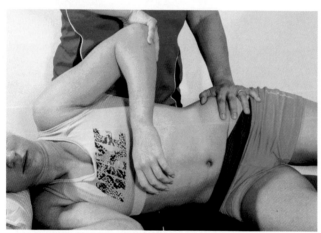

1. *Athlete is side-lying with lower leg flexed and upper leg extended (resting on plinth).*
2. *Contact athlete's ipsilateral elbow and ipsilateral iliac crest.*
3. *Abduct the shoulder, feeling for a resistance in the tissues (starting point).*
4. *Athlete actively adducts the shoulder against resistance using approximately twenty percent of overall strength for ten to twelve seconds.*
5. *Utilizing the post isometric relaxation (PIR) period (approximately twenty seconds), take the shoulder into further abduction at the same time as maintaining pelvic position with the other hand.*

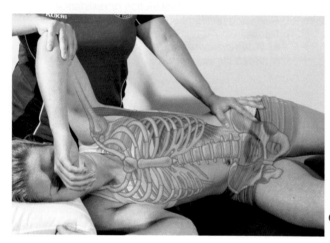

6. *Repeat these steps until no further gains are achieved.*

Thoracolumbar Fascia

The thoracolumbar fascia (TLF) consists of three separate layers:

1. Posterior (superficial to erector spinae) fibers invest medially into the spinous processes of the thoracic, lumbar, and sacral vertebrae and the associated supraspinous ligaments.
   - This layer extends from the sacrum and iliac crest to the angles of the ribs, lateral to iliocostalis
   - Latissimus dorsi partly arises from the strong membranous part of this layer.
2. The middle layer invests medially into the tissues surrounding the lumbar transverse processes and the intertransverse ligaments.
   - It extends from the lower border of the twelfth rib and lumbocostal ligament above to the iliac crest and iliolumbar ligament below
   - It lies between erector spinae and quadratus lumborum.
3. The anterior layer lies anterior to quadratus lumborum, investing into the tissues surrounding the anterior surface of the lumbar transverse processes medially.
   - Laterally it fuses with the middle layer at the lateral border of quadratus lumborum

- It extends from the iliac crest and iliolumbar ligament below to the lower border of the twelfth rib
- Superiorly it is thickened between the twelfth rib and transverse process of L1 to form the lateral arcuate ligament
- Laterally the single sheet of fascia acts as the point of attachment for transversus abdominis and the internal oblique
- In the lumbar region the thick fascia fills the space between the twelfth rib and the iliac crest, acting as a protective membrane
- In the thoracic region the fascia is thinner, sitting between erector spinae, latissimus dorsi, and the rhomboid muscles.

Action

- Multiple muscles attach to the TLF, allowing it to act as a connection point between the muscles of the lower back, pelvis, and proximal aspect of the lower extremities
- It creates stability by producing tension when these muscles contract.

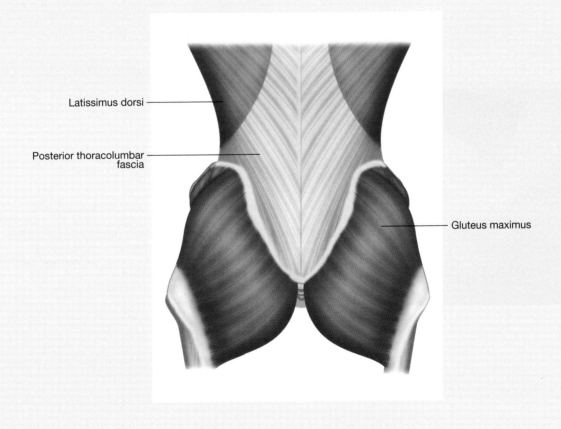

Latissimus dorsi

Posterior thoracolumbar fascia

Gluteus maximus

Figure 6.6: The thoracolumbar fascia

Soft-Tissue Treatment: Athlete Seated

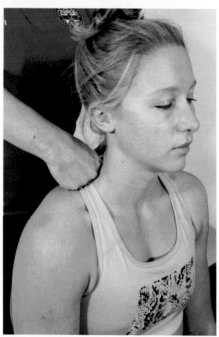

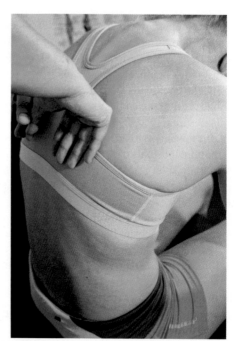

1. Athlete is seated on middle of plinth with feet placed firmly on the floor.
2. Stand behind athlete.
3. Place soft fists just anterior to the bulk of upper trapezius.

4. Maintain pressure and, when the tissues allow, slowly move the hands distally (please read Chapter 2: Fascia).

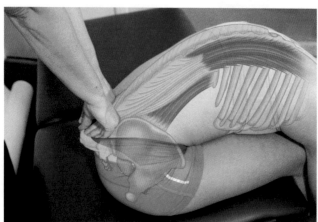

5. Maintain pressure until your hands reach the sacrum.
6. There will be areas of discomfort (pre-warn athlete).
7. There will be areas of very slow movement or periods of no movement; remain where you are until the tissues allow movement.
8. Repeat two to three times until the whole movement is fluid.

Instrument-Assisted Soft-Tissue Mobilization (IASTM): Athlete on Hands and Knees (Spine Neutral)

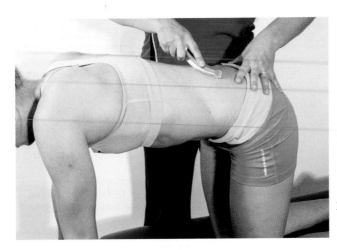

1. Initially scan the area using the long or short curve, identifying points of restriction or resistance.
    ■ Use broad strokes and slowly sweep upward, downward, obliquely, and transversely (all directions).
2. Release tension between skin and superficial fascia.
    ■ Keep pressure light.
    ■ Keep strokes swift.

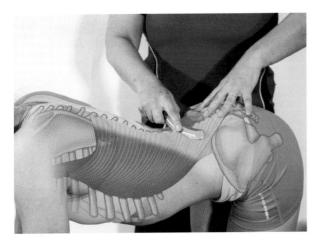
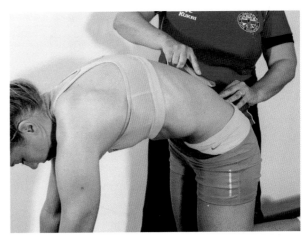

3. Instruct athlete to simultaneously flex and extend the spine.
4. Repeat sweeping, avoiding producing red bruising.

Instrument-Assisted Soft-Tissue Mobilization (IASTM): Athlete Standing

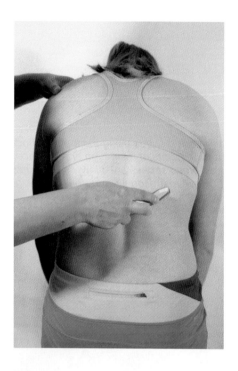

1. *Begin in neutral or slight flexion to avoid any skin slack impeding the flow of the instrument as you scan.*
2. *Scan using the short or long curves.*
   - *The short curve commonly fits well around the contours of the ribs and the lateral and posterior lumbar musculature.*
   - *The shoulder of the instrument fits well into the paraspinal groove preventing the instrument from "bumping" over the spinous processes— something which must be avoided.*
3. *Alternatively, take skin slack with your non-instrument hand.*
4. *Use broad strokes, slowly sweeping upward, downward, obliquely, and transversely (all directions).*

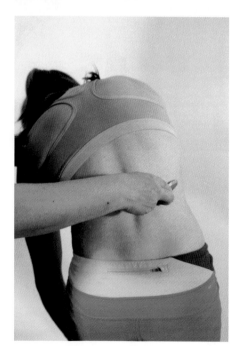

5. *When in standing:*
   - *Athlete simultaneously flexes and laterally flexes the spine.*
6. *Repeat sweeping, avoiding producing red bruising.*

Gluteus Maximus

Attachments

- Gluteal surface of the ilium behind the posterior gluteal line
- Posterior border of the ilium and adjacent part of the iliac crest
- Arises from the side of the coccyx and posterior aspect of the sacrum
- Upper part of the sacrotuberous ligament
- Upper fibers invest into aponeurosis of the sacrospinalis
- Deep anterior fibers arise from the fascia covering gluteus medius
- Fibers pass downward and forward toward the upper part of the femur
- Superficial fibers (approximately three-quarters) form a separate lamina that narrows down and invests between the two layers of the fascia lata, helping to form the iliotibial tract
- The deeper fibers (one-quarter) form a broad aponeurosis that invests into the periosteum of the gluteal tuberosity of the femur.

Innervation

- Inferior gluteal nerve (root value L5, S1, and S2)
- The skin covering the muscle (branches from L2 and L3).

Action

- Pulls the shaft of the femur backward, producing extension of the flexed hip joint
- Lower fibers nearer to lateral side of thigh rotate the thigh laterally during extension
- Lower fibers can adduct the thigh
- Upper fibers may help in abduction
- Fibers investing into the iliotibial tract can produce extension of the knee
- If the femur is fixed, contraction of the gluteus maximus pulls the ilium and pelvis backward around the hip joint (lifting the trunk from a flexed position)
- With the hamstrings the GM raises the trunk from a flexed position
- Balances pelvis on the femoral heads (maintaining upright posture)
- Aids lateral rotation of the femur when standing (raising longitudinal arch of the foot)
- Stepping up onto box, climbing, running.

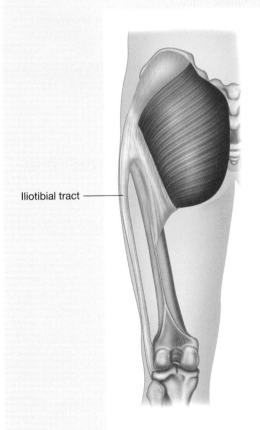

Iliotibial tract

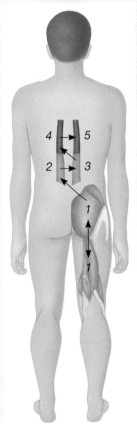

Muscle activation sequence:
1. *Hamstrings & gluteus maximus*
2. *Contralateral lumbar extensors*
3. *Ipsilateral lumbar extensors*
4. *Contralateral thoracolumbar extensors*
5. *Ipsilateral thoracolumbar extensors*

Figure 6.7: Gluteus maximus (GM)

Figure 6.8: Hip extension firing pattern

Gluteus Maximus (GM)

The GM is a powerful extensor that works reciprocally with the hamstrings during the gait cycle. Weakness of this muscle has a direct effect on the function/stabilization of the posterior sling and SIJ (early- and midstance phases) as well as increasing activation of the hamstring group (leading to hypertonicity and potential injury). Inhibition also leads to compensation (latissimus dorsi activation/hypertonicity), altering function throughout the body (e.g. shoulder position).

In addition, the GM and psoas have a reciprocal relationship: Inhibition of the GM may lead to an overactive or hypertonic psoas (assess the length). Hypertonicity of GM may lead to inactivity/inhibition of the psoas. This knowledge is important when clinically reasoning why the presenting SIJ is struggling to attain/maintain optimal function.

The ideal extension pattern is achieved when all the muscles involved fire in a predetermined optimal sequence (see figure 6.8):

- GM or the hamstring group may activate first
- Contralateral lumbar erector spinae then ipsilateral lumbar erector spinae
- Contralateral thoracolumbar erector spinae then ipsilateral thoracolumbar erector spinae.

If overactivation or underactivation of a particular muscle group is detected, pelvic position can be affected along with excessive hyperextension of the lumbar vertebrae (hyperlordosis).

Palpation

1. Athlete is prone.
2. Palpate along the lateral edge of the sacrum until you reach the coccyx.
3. Palpate from the posterior superior iliac spine (PSIS) to approximately two inches along the posterior surface of the iliac crest.
4. Palpate the gluteal tuberosity.
5. Palpate all of the tissue between these points, checking for taut bands and hypertonic tissues.
6. To confirm location, athlete extends hip.

Assessment for Length

1. Athlete is supine with hips and knees flexed.
2. Pelvis in neutral.
3. Flex athlete's thigh toward the pelvis without initiating posterior pelvic tilt (sacrum flat on plinth).
   - If sacrum lifts off the plinth, stop the movement and note the range
   - This indicates short GM.
4. Reassess after treatment.

Assessment for Strength

1. Athlete is standing, with trunk flexed over plinth.
2. Athlete flexes knee and extends hip.
3. Stabilize athlete's pelvis, preventing hyperextension of the lumbar spine.
4. Athlete extends the hip against your resistance (proximal to knee joint).
5. This is graded:
   - 5/5—strong contraction (normal)
   - 4/5—firm contraction (good)
   - 3/5—soft contraction (fair)
   - 2/5—slight contraction (poor)
   - 1/5—flicker (trace)
   - 0/5—no contraction detected.
6. Weakness may be due to inhibition, trigger points, pain, or muscle length.
7. Reassess after treatment.

Gluteus Medius and Minimus

Gluteus Medius Attachments

- Emerges from the gluteal aponeurosis and the outer surface of tissues covering the ilium (between the iliac crest and the greater trochanter)
- Covered with a strong layer of fascia, sharing the posterior part with gluteus maximus
- Overlapped by the gluteus maximus
- Posterior fibers pass downward and forward
- Middle fibers pass straight downward
- Anterior fibers pass downward and backward
- Fibers converge into a flattened tendon that invests into the periosteum and fascial tissues of other structures surrounding the greater trochanter
- The tendon passes downward and forward and is separated from the trochanter by a bursa.

Gluteus Medius Innervation

- Superior gluteal nerve (root value L4, L5, and S1)
- Skin covering (L1 and L2).

Action

- Pelvis fixed—pulls the greater trochanter upward and the femoral shaft laterally (abduction), and aids medial rotation of the femur
- Lower attachment fixed—pulls down the ilium ipsilaterally (downward tilt of the pelvis), thereby producing upward tilt contralaterally
- Femur fixed—rotates the contralateral pelvis forward
- Vital role in walking, running, and single-leg weight bearing

- Supports and slightly lifts the weight-bearing pelvis when the contralateral leg is taken off the ground, allowing the limb to be placed anteriorly for the next step
- If these mechanics are dysfunctional/inhibited the pelvis drops instead (Trendelenberg sign), making walking difficult and running virtually impossible.

Gluteus Minimus Attachments

- Has the largest investment into the gluteal surface of the ilium
- In front of the anterior and above the inferior gluteal lines
- Fibers pass downward, backward, and slightly laterally to form a tendon
- The tendon invests into the tissues surrounding the anterosuperior surface of the greater trochanter.

Gluteus Minimus Innervation

- Superior gluteal nerve (root value L4, L5, and S1)
- Skin covering (L1).

Action

- Upper portion fixed—anterior fibers medially rotate the femur
- Lower portion fixed—raises the contralateral pelvis (similar to gluteus medius)
- Pulls anterior ilium forward, swinging the contralateral pelvis forward
- Supports and controls pelvic movements when walking and running (when contralateral leg is off the ground).

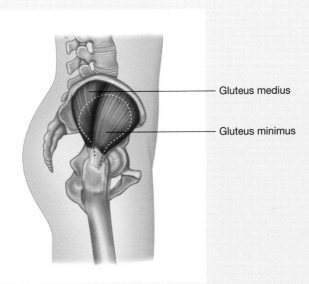

Gluteus medius

Gluteus minimus

Figure 6.9: Gluteus medius and gluteus minimus

Palpation

1. Athlete is side-lying.
2. Locate anterior superior iliac spine (ASIS) and PSIS.
3. Tissues sit just below the iliac crest and between these landmarks.
4. Palpate tissues from just below the iliac crest to the greater trochanter (sink in deeper to locate minimus).
5. To confirm location, athlete abducts hip.

Assessment for Length

1. Athlete is side-lying, lower hip and knee flexed.
2. Upper hip and knee extended.
   - Is the limb resting on the plinth?
   - No—indicative of short gluteus medius and minimus or tensor fascia lata.
3. Reassess after treatment.

Assessment for Strength

1. Athlete is side-lying, with lower hip and knee flexed.
2. Upper hip and knee extended should be resting on plinth.
3. Athlete abducts the hip.
   - No flexion or lateral rotation is permitted.
4. Stabilize athlete's pelvis and provide resistance proximal to the knee joint.
5. This is graded:
   - 5/5—strong contraction (normal)
   - 4/5—firm contraction (good)
   - 3/5—soft contraction (fair)
   - 2/5—slight contraction (poor)
   - 1/5—flicker (trace)
   - 0/5— No contraction detected.
6. Weakness may be due to inhibition, trigger points, pain, or muscle length.
7. Reassess after treatment.

Soft-Tissue Treatment: Athlete Prone

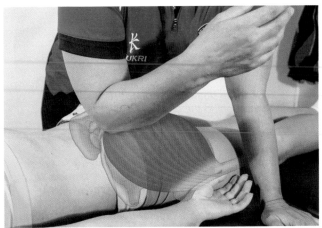

1. Using your elbow, slowly melt into the tissues just lateral to the PSIS, using a VAS score of 6/10.
2. Maintain the pressure until the VAS score reduces to approximately 2/10.
3. Athlete tilts the ipsilateral ilium caudad (downward toward the feet).
4. Following the direction of the fibers (downward and forward), repeat this process every inch or so until you approach the greater trochanter.
5. Return to approximately one inch below your starting position and repeat this process along the lateral border of the sacrum on the ipsilateral side.
6. Trigger points can be treated here with either ischemic compression or dry-needling techniques.

Soft-Tissue Treatment: Athlete Supine

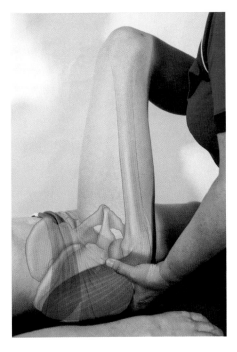

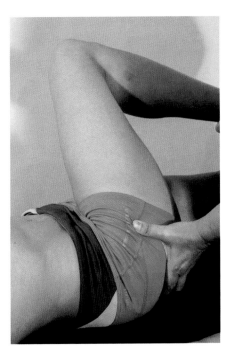

1. Stand on the side of the athlete to be treated.
2. The athlete's hip and knee are flexed and passively taken up so that the foot is no longer resting on the table.
3. Engage the tissue around the greater trochanter with soft thumbs as the hip is passively adducted (slowly).

Soft-Tissue Treatment: Athlete Side-Lying 1

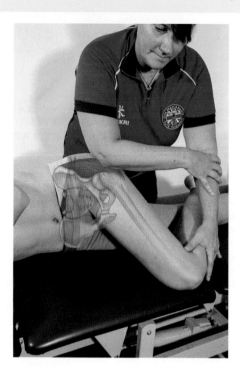

1. *Side to be treated is uppermost.*
2. *Stand behind the athlete.*
3. *The athlete's uppermost hip and knee are flexed to ninety degrees, with the knee resting on the plinth in front.*
4. *With skin-to-skin contact (if possible; if not, through thin clothing is acceptable, particularly when trackside) sink your elbow into the tissues surrounding the greater trochanter.*
5. *Starting above the greater trochanter and moving in an anticlockwise direction, gently sink into the tissues surrounding the greater trochanter.*
6. *As you sense the tissue giving in the area being treated, move to the next location and repeat until the tissues surrounding the trochanter circumference have been covered.*

Soft-Tissue Treatment: Athlete Side-Lying 2

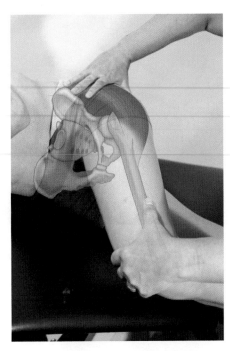

1. *Stand facing the athlete.*
2. *The athlete's uppermost leg is hip flexed to ninety degrees and knee flexed to ninety degrees, with the foot placed on your hip.*
3. *Holding areas of the muscle belly between your fingers and thumbs, passively flex the hip by stepping forward.*
   - *Facilitate the movement by following with the contact hand (pressure maintained)—good for painful movements initially.*
   - *Resist the movement by locking into the tissues, maintaining that position whilst the tissues are actively or passively taken into position.*

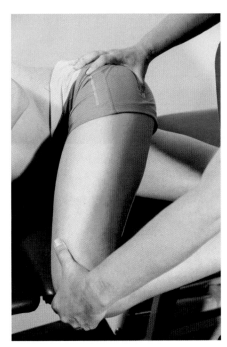

4. *Follow with soft thumbs one to one and a half inches distally off the posterior aspect of the greater trochanter, around the distal attachment (gluteal tuberosity).*

5. *Take the hip into deeper flexion then add an adduction force by slowly pushing down on the lateral aspect of the knee.*

Soft-Tissue Treatment: Athlete Side-Lying 3

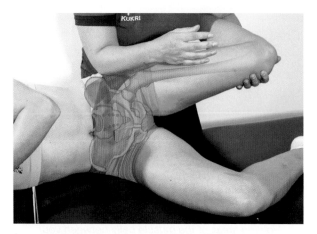

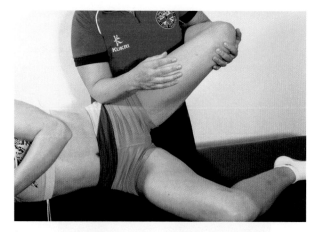

1. *Athlete has both knees and hips flexed.*
2. *Contact the bulk of gluteus medius and minimus with your elbow and hold the athlete's knee with the other hand.*

3. *Passively abduct the upper hip with the hand holding the knee, and sink slowly into the tissues with the elbow.*
4. *Maintain this contact and depth.*

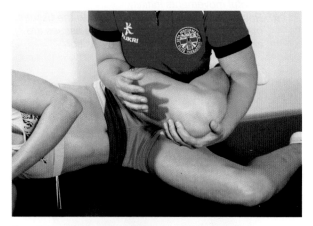

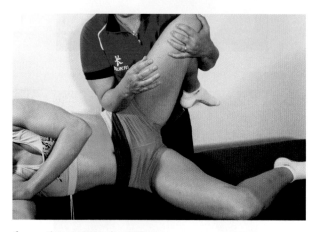

5. *Take the hip slowly into adduction and flexion (this can be painful—remember your VAS).*

6. *...then external rotation,*

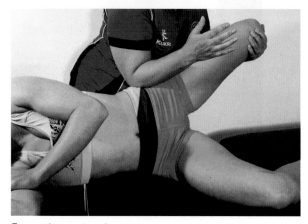

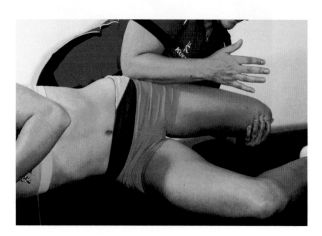

7. *...then extension,*

8. *...then adduction.*

Soft-Tissue Treatment: Athlete Side-Lying 4

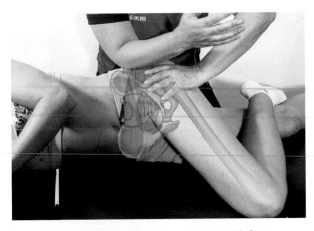

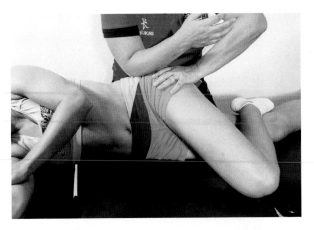

1. Athlete's upper leg has knee flexed, with foot resting on extended lower leg.
2. Contact the bulk of gluteus medius and minimus with your elbow.

3. Athlete abducts hip and raises the knee off the plinth slightly.

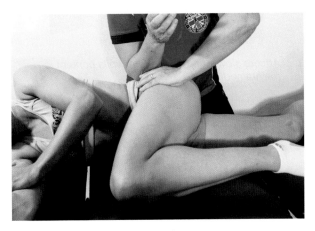

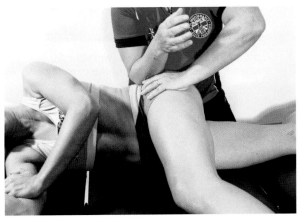

4. Athlete flexes hip toward chest.

5. Athlete extends the knee in this position.

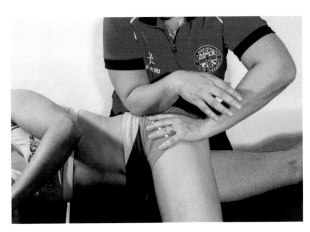

6. Athlete adducts the extended leg over the edge of the plinth.

Soft-Tissue Treatment: Athlete Standing

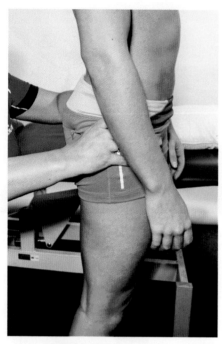

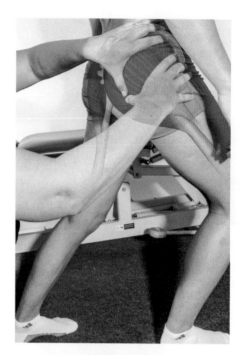

1. *Contact the bulk of the glutes with your flat thumbs and work into different areas of the muscle belly.*

2. *Athlete slowly lunges forward while contact is maintained.*

Dry Needling for Glutes

Dry needling should only be performed by a qualified and insured physical therapist, owing to the invasive nature of the technique and serious anatomical considerations.

Gluteus Maximus

1. Athlete is prone/side-lying.
2. Note the referral pattern—does this represent your athlete's pain?
3. Palpate the tissues for taut bands.
4. Insert the needle perpendicularly through the skin and into the taut band.
5. Avoid penetrating the sciatic nerve (imperative that you know your anatomy).

Gluteus Medius or Gluteus Minimus

1. Athlete is prone/supine/side-lying.
2. Note referral pattern—does this represent your athlete's pain?
3. Palpate the tissues for taut bands.
4. Insert the needle perpendicularly through the skin and into the taut band along the curve of the iliac crest (bone/periosteum tapping is common).
5. Avoid penetrating the sciatic nerve and superior gluteal blood vessels.

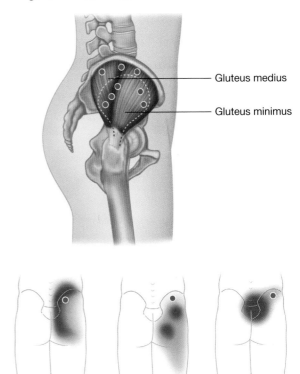

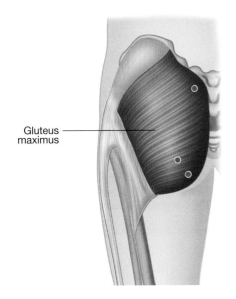

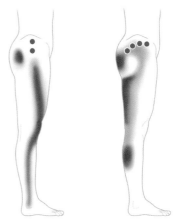

Figure 6.11: Gluteus medius trigger points and referral pattern

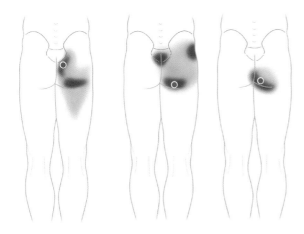

Figure 6.10: Gluteus maximus trigger points (referral common to SIJ)

Figure 6.12: Gluteus minimus trigger points and referral pattern

Muscle Energy Techniques (MET): Athlete Supine 1

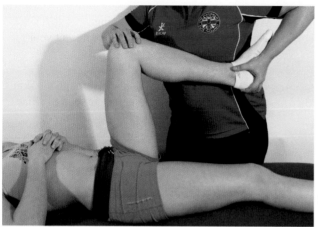

1. Athlete's hip and knee are flexed and taken to the position where resistance is first detected (starting point) or where the sacrum lifts away from the plinth.
2. Athlete actively extends the hip against resistance using approximately twenty percent of overall strength for ten to twelve seconds.

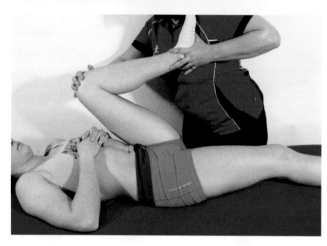

3. Utilizing the PIR period (approximately twenty seconds), take the femur into further flexion whilst maintaining the contralateral femur position with the other hand.
4. Repeat these steps until no further gains are achieved.

Muscle Energy Techniques (MET): Athlete Supine 2

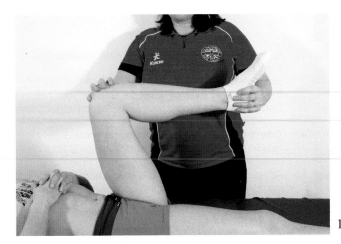

1. *Athlete's hip and knee are flexed.*

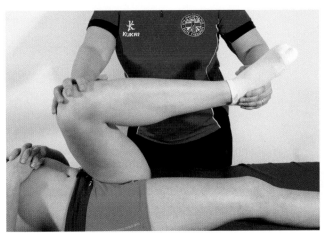

2. *Take femur into adduction to the position where resistance is first detected (starting point).*
3. *Athlete actively abducts and externally rotates the hip against resistance using approximately twenty percent of overall strength for ten to twelve seconds.*

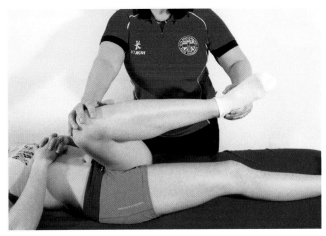

4. *Utilizing the PIR period (approximately twenty seconds), take the femur into further adduction whilst maintaining the contralateral pelvic position with the other hand.*
5. *Repeat these steps until no further gains are achieved.*

Muscle Energy Techniques (MET): Athlete Supine 3

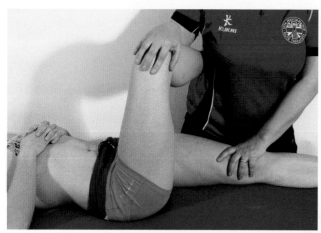

1. Athlete's hip is flexed and externally rotated, and knee is flexed.
2. Stand on the opposite side, and place the foot of the flexed and externally rotated hip on your hip.
3. Contact athlete's ipsilateral knee (lateral aspect) and contralateral femur.
4. Take the femur into further external rotation and flexion to the position where resistance is first detected (starting point).
5. Athlete actively extends and medially rotates the hip against resistance using approximately twenty percent of their overall strength for ten to twelve seconds.

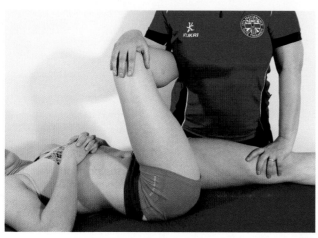

6. Utilizing the PIR period (approximately twenty seconds), take the femur into further flexion and external rotation whilst maintaining the contralateral femur position with the other hand.
7. Repeat these steps until no further gains are achieved.

Posterior Pelvic Ligaments

Posterior Sacroiliac Ligaments

- Lay behind and above the SIJ, and are thicker and stronger than those anteriorly
- Superficial to the interosseous ligament and the SIJ
- Consist of numerous bands passing between the sacrum and the ilium
- Longer fibers fan obliquely downward and medially
- Upper portion (short posterior sacroiliac ligament) passes horizontally between the first and second transverse tubercles of the sacrum and the iliac tuberosity
  - *Resisting forward movement of the sacrum*
- Long posterior sacroiliac ligament is the most superficial, running almost vertically from PSIS to the third and fourth transverse tubercles of the sacrum
  - *Resists downward movement of the sacrum with respect to the ilium.*

Iliolumbar Ligaments

- Pass inferiorly and laterally from the tissue surrounding the transverse process of L5, and sometimes L4, to the tissue surrounding the posterior inner lip of the iliac crest

- In reality it is the thickened lower border of the anterior and middle layers of the TLF.

Sacrotuberous Ligaments

- The STL is a flat triangular band
- It attaches superiorly to the posterior border of the ilium between the posterior superior and posterior inferior iliac spines to the ipsilateral posterolateral sacrum distal the auricular surface and to the superolateral part of the coccyx
- Fibers travel downward and laterally toward the ischial tuberosity, converging as they do so
- Here, the fibers twist upon themselves then diverge again so that the attachment is along the lower margin of the ischial ramus
- The most superficial fibers invest into the ischial tuberosity, where they blend with the fibers of the biceps femoris
- The posterior surface of the ligament gives attachment to GM
- The STL provides stability to the sacrum on the innominate by preventing forward tilting.

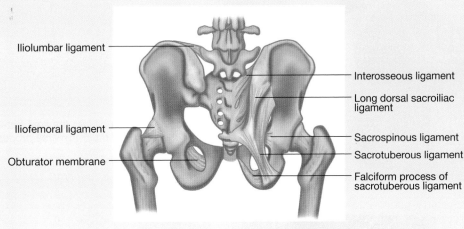

Figure 6.13: Posterior pelvic ligaments

Labels: Iliolumbar ligament; Iliofemoral ligament; Obturator membrane; Interosseous ligament; Long dorsal sacroiliac ligament; Sacrospinous ligament; Sacrotuberous ligament; Falciform process of sacrotuberous ligament

Palpation of the Iliolumbar and Sacroiliac Ligaments

1. With the athlete prone, locate the PSIS, L4, and L5.
2. Slide your fingers between the PSIS and the transverse processes of L4/L5.
3. Sink slowly through the fascial tissue of the lumbar fascia.
4. You may be able to detect the taut, slightly oblique fibers of the ligament.

Palpation of the Sacrotuberous Ligaments

1. With the athlete prone, locate the ischial tuberosity and the lateral border of the sacrum.
2. Slide your fingers from the ischial tuberosity to the edge of the sacrum.
3. Between these two points you should be able to palpate the broad solid ligament.

Soft-Tissue Treatment: Athlete Prone

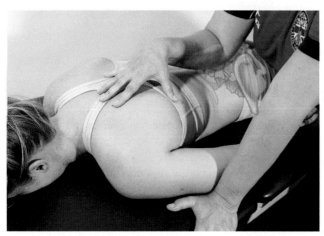

1. *Palpate the area around the lower lumbar vertebrae and the iliac crests for hypertonicity/tissue tension/ tissue resistance.*
2. *Place the tip of your elbow into the area between the edge of the ilium and the transverse process of L4 (VAS 6/10 maximum).*
3. *Sink slowly into the tissue and wait until some of the tension is reduced (VAS 2/10), then lay your forearm parallel to the spinous processes with your hand facing in a cephalad direction (toward the head).*
4. *Maintaining this depth, and once the tissues allow, move very slowly toward the area between the coccyx and the ischial tuberosity—staying along the lateral sacral crest.*
   - *This can be tender (pre-warn athlete).*
5. *Repeat on the other side.*

Soft-Tissue Treatment: Athlete Side-Lying (Iliolumbar and Sacroiliac Ligaments)

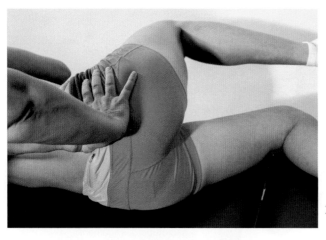

1. *Place your thumbs into the area between the edge of the ilium and the transverse process of L4 (VAS 6/10 maximum).*
2. *Sink slowly into the tissue and wait until some of the tension is reduced (VAS 2/10).*

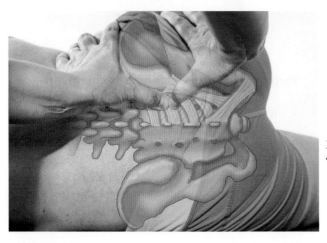

3. *Instruct the athlete to slowly flex the ipsilateral hip.*
4. *Move thumbs slightly (to address fascia investing into these ligaments):*
   - *Above the initial area*
     - *Athlete is instructed to flex the ipsilateral hip*
   - *Below the initial area*
     - *Athlete is instructed to flex the ipsilateral hip.*

Soft-Tissue Treatment: Athlete Side-Lying (Sacrotuberous Ligaments)

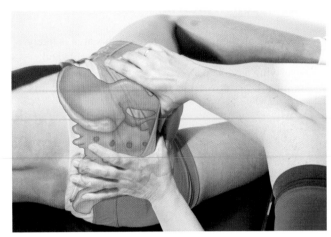

1. *Athlete has lower leg flexed for balance, and upper leg extended.*
2. *Place your thumbs into the area between the medial border of the sacrum and the ischial tuberosity (VAS 6/10 maximum).*
3. *Sink slowly into the tissue and wait until some of the tension is reduced (VAS 2/10).*
4. *Athlete flexes hip and takes hold of knee to pull into further flexion.*
5. *Repeat points 1–4 above until all tissues are covered (working distally) between the medial border of the sacrum and the ischial tuberosity.*

Soft-Tissue Treatment: Athlete Standing (Sacrotuberous Ligaments)

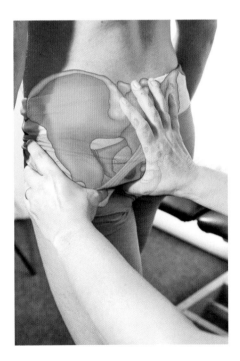

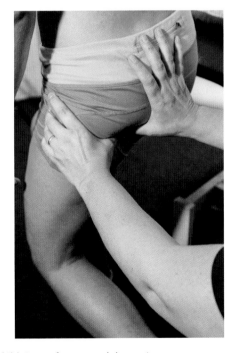

1. *Athlete stands with small-stride stance.*
2. *The side to be treated should be the posterior stance leg.*
3. *Sink into the tissues lying between the edge of the sacrum and the ischial tuberosity.*
4. *Maintain pressure and direction:*
   - *Travelling with the tissues to facilitate the movement.*
   - *Blocking movement by maintaining "lock" to facilitate a stretch of the tissues.*

5. *Athlete performs a mini squat.*
6. *Repeat until all tissues have been addressed between the two points.*

Dry Needling for Posterior Pelvic Ligaments

Dry needling should only be performed by a qualified and insured physical therapist, owing to the invasive nature of the technique and serious anatomical considerations.

1. Athlete is prone.
2. Locate the ligaments (see Palpation, page 97).
3. Multiple needles can be placed perpendicularly or at an angle to avoid piercing the foramina.
4. Care must be taken so as not to pierce the medial cluneal nerves (sacroiliac ligament).
5. Care must be taken so as not to pierce the lower superior cluneal nerve (iliolumbar ligament).
6. Needle is placed in an inferior and lateral direction.

Instrument-Assisted Soft-Tissue Mobilization (IASTM)

Working on the fascial structures in this area is likely to have an impact on the posterior SIJ capsule and overlying associated fascial structures (superficial lamina of the TLF, lateral raphe, gluteus medius, and gluteus maximus).

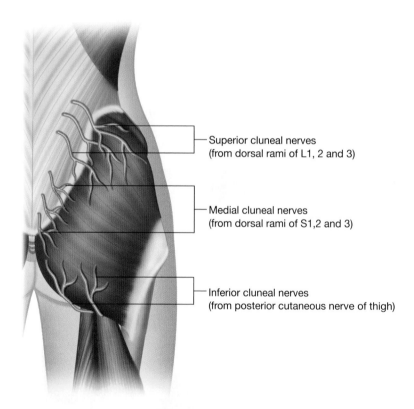

Superior cluneal nerves
(from dorsal rami of L1, 2 and 3)

Medial cluneal nerves
(from dorsal rami of S1,2 and 3)

Inferior cluneal nerves
(from posterior cutaneous nerve of thigh)

Figure 6.14: Anatomy of the cluneal nerves

Instrument-Assisted Soft-Tissue Mobilization (IASTM): Athlete Side-Lying

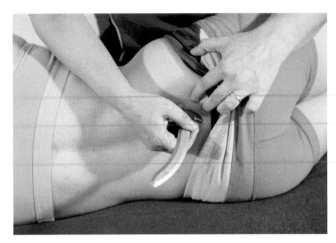

1. *Scan the area surrounding the SIJ looking for restrictions.*
2. *Contact using the flat edge.*
3. *Utilize the "beak" without losing contact.*

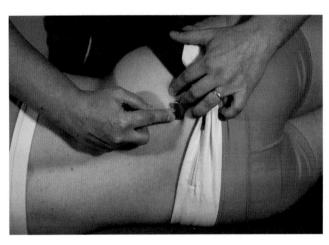

4. *Athlete flexes the hip and returns to starting position.*
5. *You can facilitate this movement if necessary.*

Instrument-Assisted Soft-Tissue Mobilization (IASTM): Athlete Four-Point Kneeling

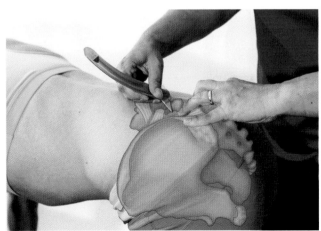

1. *Use small strokes, slowly sweeping in different directions (using the flat edge) over the surface of the tissues covering the ligaments. Later use the beak to pick between the ligaments.*
2. *Athlete simultaneously tilts pelvis forward and backward.*
3. *Repeat the broad sweeps, avoiding producing red bruising.*

Biceps Femoris

Attachments

- Situated on the posterolateral aspect of the thigh
- Arises by two heads which are separated by a considerable distance
- Long head—attaches to the lower medial facet on the ischial tuberosity with the tendon of the semitendinosus spreading into the sacrotuberous ligament
- These two tendons descend for a short distance then separate into the two individual muscles
- The long head of biceps femoris forms a fusiform muscle running downwards and laterally across the posterior aspect of the thigh superficial to the sciatic nerve
- In the lower third of the thigh the long head narrows and is joined on its deep aspect by the short head of biceps femoris
- The short head has its upper attachments from the lower half of the lateral lip of the linea aspera reaching almost as far up as the attachment of the gluteus maximus and running down onto the upper half of the lateral supracondylar line of the femur
- Some fibers of the short head gradually blend with the narrowing tendon of the long head which lies superficial to it
- The tendon crosses the posterolateral aspect of the knee and runs towards the fibula
- Prior to attaching to the periosteum surrounding the head of the fibula, the tendon of biceps femoris is split into two by the fibular (lateral) collateral ligament
- Some fibers of the tendon join the ligament, while a few others attach to the periosteum surrounding the lateral tibial condyle and some to the posterior aspect of the lateral intermuscular septum, which lies just in front of it
- A bursa separates the tendon from the lateral collateral ligament.

Innervation

- The long head is supplied by the tibial division of the sciatic nerve
- The short head is supplied by the common (fibular) peroneal division (root value of both L5, S1–2)
- Skin covering the muscle (root S2).

Action

- Helps the other two hamstrings extend the hip joint particularly when the trunk is flexed and is to be raised to the erect position
- All three hamstrings work eccentrically to control forward flexion of the trunk

- Aids the other hamstrings when flexing the knee joint
- With the knee in a semiflexed position rotates the tibia laterally on the femur
- If the foot is fixed rotates the femur and pelvis medially on the tibia.

Functional Activity of the Hamstrings

- Flexion of the knee and their stabilizing effect is a very important function
- Holding the trunk in a flexed position (starting blocks) and raising the trunk from a flexed position requires a great deal of power and this mode of action may well be why the hamstrings are so frequently injured (the first 10–20m of sprinting)
- Also play an important part in the fine balance of the pelvis when standing, particularly when the upper trunk is being moved from vertical
- Working in conjunction with the abdominal muscles, anterosuperiorly and the gluteus maximus posteroinferiorly, the anterosuperior tilt of the pelvis can be altered having an affect on lumbar lordosis
- Have a role in decelerating the forward motion of the tibia when the free swinging leg is extended during walking (preventing the knee from snapping into extension).

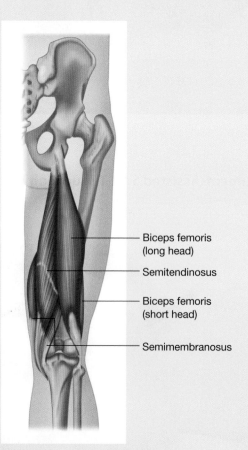

Biceps femoris (long head)

Semitendinosus

Biceps femoris (short head)

Semimembranosus

Figure 6.15: Posterior thigh muscles

Palpation

1. Athlete prone.
2. Palpate the proximal aspect from the common attachment around the ischium to the distal attachment around the head of the fibula.
3. Athlete resists knee flexion.

Assessment for Length 1

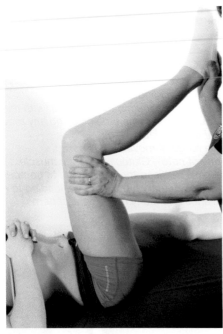

1. *Athlete in supine with arms across the chest.*
2. *The ipsilateral hip is passively flexed (knee flexed) to ninety degrees while the contralateral leg remains fully extended and resting on the plinth.*
3. *Foot held by the therapist remains fully relaxed.*

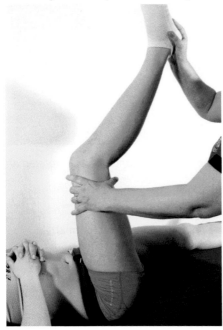 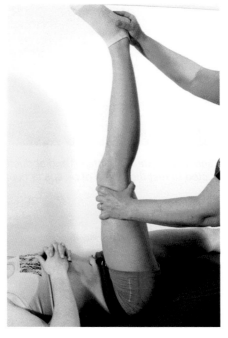

4. *Therapist passively extends the knee, keeping the hip in ninety degrees of flexion.*
5. *The angle between the femur and tibia are noted.*

Assessment for Length 2

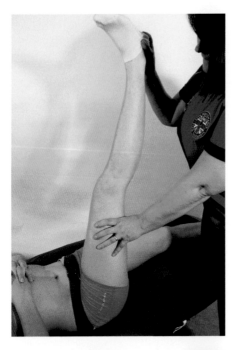

1. *Athlete supine with hands placed behind their back to prevent excessive posterior tilt of the pelvis (can give a false reading of flexibility).*
2. *Therapist flexes the hip to be tested (with the knee extended) at the same time blocking any movement from the contralateral leg.*
   - *the range of movement is noted.*
3. *Worthy of note—Gluteus maximus muscle weakness can lead the hamstrings to compensate and act as primary hip extensors, leading to muscle imbalance and faulty movement patterns.*

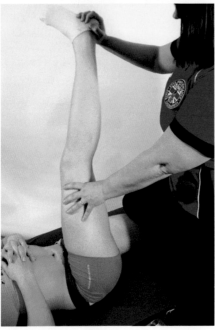

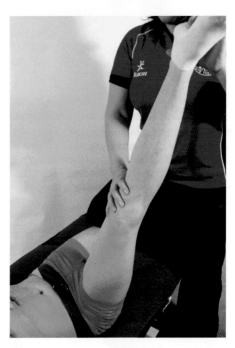

4. *Hip should be externally rotated and abducted to test length of medial hamstrings and internally rotated and adducted to test the length of biceps femoris.*

Assessment for Strength

1. Athlete prone.
2. Knee flexed to varying degrees (90, 45, 10) and held in that position while therapist attempts to extend the knee.
   - No compensatory patterns are allowed
   - No lifting or rotation of the hips, thorax or shoulders
   - No use of the arms.

3. This is graded:
   - 5/5—strong contraction (normal)
   - 4/5—firm contraction (good)
   - 3/5—soft contraction (fair)
   - 2/5—slight contraction (poor)
   - 1/5—flicker (trace)
   - 0/5— No contraction detected.

Soft-Tissue Treatment: Athlete Supine

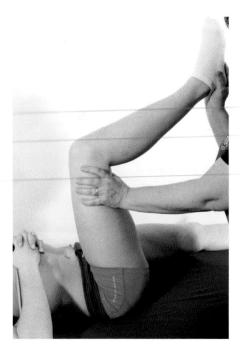
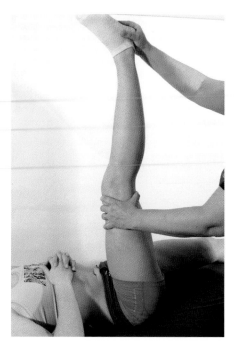

1. *Hip and knee flexed to ninety degrees.*
2. *Using the flat edge of your thumb, slowly melt into the tissues of the biceps femoris belly. Using a VAS score of 6/10.*
3. *Maintain the pressure until the VAS score reduces to approximately 2/10.*

4. *Passively extend the knee and repeat this process travelling towards the ischium.*
5. *Repeat points 2 and 3, except this time ask the athlete to straighten their knee actively, lock into the tissues as before, and wait for the VAS to reduce to approximately 2/10.*
6. *Ask the athlete to add internal and external rotation of the hip.*

Muscle Energy Techniques (MET): Hamstrings 1—Athlete Supine

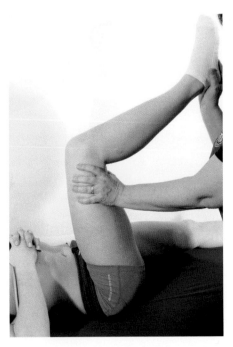

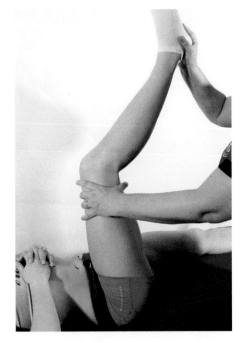

1. *Assess straight-leg raise (SLR) for range (quality and quantity).*
2. *Athlete is supine with legs extended.*
3. *Take the side to be treated into the Lasègue test position (hip and knee flexed).*
4. *Passively flex the athlete's hip to ninety degrees while the ipsilateral calf rests on your shoulder in the position where you first detected resistance.*

5. *Hold the femur in place with both hands placed just proximal to the knee joint.*
6. *Athlete flexes the knee against your resistance using approximately twenty percent of overall strength for ten to twelve seconds.*

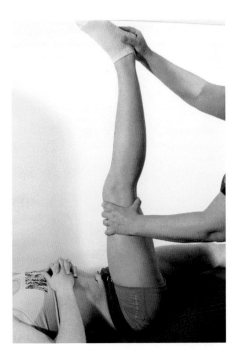

7. *Utilizing the PIR period (approximately twenty seconds), take the ipsilateral knee further into extension.*
8. *Repeat these steps until no further gains are achieved.*

Muscle Energy Techniques (MET): Hamstrings 2—Athlete Supine

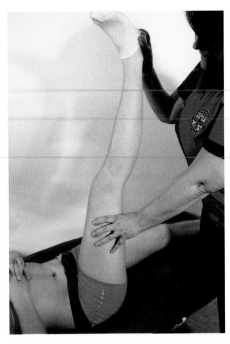
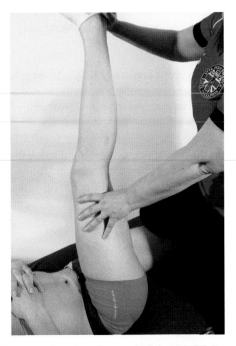

1. *Assess straight-leg raise (SLR) for range (quality and quantity) (good to place arms behind back to prevent sacral movement affecting range of movement).*
2. *Athlete is supine with legs extended.*
3. *Passively flex the athlete's hip to where you feel resistance (hamstring group).*
   - *Hip flexed, abducted and externally rotated (medial hamstrings).*
   - *Hip flexed, adducted and internally rotated (biceps femoris).*

4. *Place one hand on the contralateral ASIS for stabilization (or resist femoral flexion).*
5. *Either hold the ipsilateral leg with the other hand, or place it on your shoulder.*
6. *Athlete extends hip against your resistance, using approximately twenty percent of overall strength for ten to twelve seconds.*
7. *Utilizing the PIR period (approximately twenty seconds), take the ipsilateral femur further into flexion.*
8. *Repeat these steps until no further gains are achieved.*

Dry Needling for Hamstrings

Dry needling should only be performed by a qualified and insured physical therapist owing to the invasive nature of the technique and serious anatomical considerations

1. Athlete in prone and completely relaxed (pillow can be placed under the lower leg).
2. Note referral pattern—does this represent your athletes pain?
3. Palpate the biceps femoris for taut bands
4. Insert the needle perpendicularly through the skin and into the taut band or painful area.
5. Avoid penetrating the sciatic nerve (imperative that you know your anatomy).

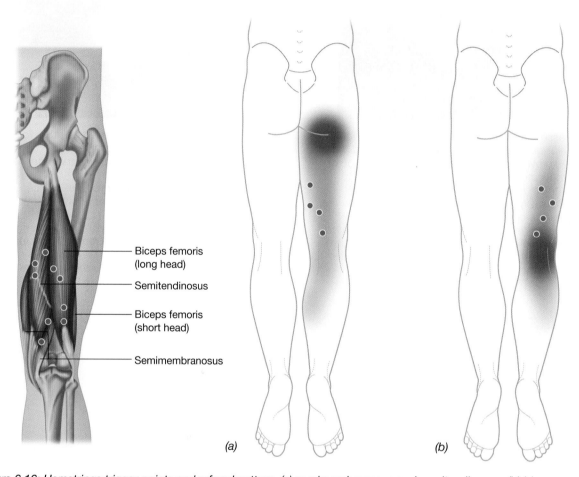

- Biceps femoris (long head)
- Semitendinosus
- Biceps femoris (short head)
- Semimembranosus

(a) (b)

Figure 6.16: Hamstrings trigger points and referral pattern, (a) semimembranosus and semitendinosus, (b) biceps femoris

Dynamic Taping of the Posterior Oblique Sling

Aims

- To resist flexion movement at the hip and trunk to reduce the workload requirements placed upon GM and erector spine and being compensated for by excessive activity of biceps femoris, or to reduce maladaptive, rigid "splinting" strategies by providing some of the force generation and load dissipation externally
- To resist loss of the lumbar lordosis to maintain sacral nutation and therefore more effective form closure, force closure, and load transfer
- To assist the action of the posterior oblique sling of GM, TLF, and contralateral latissimus dorsi
- To initiate the recovery of extension from a flexed position of the spine.

Equipment

- Three-inch Dynamic Tape®, Dynamic Tape® Adhesive Spray.

Athlete's Position

- Prone on elbows with sacral nutation and scapula retraction and depression
- The technique may be applied in standing if the patient has a lot of difficulty getting up and down from a lying position.

Line of Pull

- Start on the scapula.
- Pass inferiorly and obliquely to cross the low lumbar spine and the contralateral SIJ.
- Continue inferiorly down the midline of the thigh to assist the hip extension component.
- Repeat on the other side.
- The tapes should cross at the low lumbar region and will therefore resist the loss of lumbar lordosis.

Re-evaluation

- Lumbar flexion and recovery of extension, particularly if a reversal of the lumbopelvic rhythm was previously present, indicating poor ability to transfer load with a normal movement pattern.

Note

- Lightly spray the back of the first layer with adhesive spray before applying the second layer.

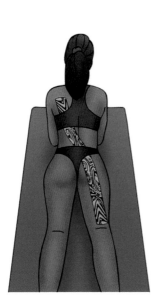
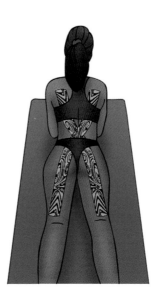
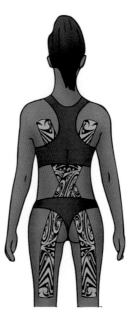

Figure 6.17: Diagrams showing taping over clothing for dignity; however the tape must be attached to the skin. This is much easier if the athlete is asked to wear small underwear—the tape can then be passed beneath the underwear and fixed to the skin.

Dynamic Taping for Pelvic Closure

Aim
- To provide an external pelvic compressive force to augment force closure and in turn improve timing and activation of GM and biceps femoris muscles.

Equipment
- Two- or three-inch Dynamic Tape®, depending on the size of the patient and force generation requirements
- A double-layer PowerBand may be required to generate sufficient force.

Position
- Generally apply with patient standing with increased lumbar lordosis to create sacral nutation.

Line of Pull
- The tape should be positioned just proximal to the greater trochanters, on the wing of the pelvis, and continue circumferentially (finish on skin to improve adhesion) to create a compressive effect.

Re-evaluation
- Reassess the active straight-leg raise or other functional tasks that had demonstrated poor load-transfer capacity (e.g. single-leg standing, stairs).

Dynamic Taping to Reduce Load on Posterior Ligamentous Structures

Aim
- To provide a posterior compressive force to reduce load on posterior ligamentous structures, which have been shown to increase uptake with SIJ incompetence
- To resist counternutation and encourage maintenance of lumbar lordosis to permit effective form and force closure, and resist lumbar flexion moment to assist lumbar multifidus/erector spinae function
- To aid in hip flexion and internal rotation control (particularly on the weight-bearing limb) to assist the weak, delayed, yet overactive GM and the overloaded, compensatory activity of biceps femoris
- May provide a firm backboard against which pressure can be developed owing to contraction and swelling of the muscular elements thereby augmenting stability.

Equipment
- Two- and three-inch Dynamic Tape®.

Position
- Patient prone, lying, or on elbows with sacral nutation.

Line of Pull
- Pelvic strips should start on ASIS, pass directly over the SIJ, behind the axis of the contralateral hip (to assist extension and resist flexion) and finish anterior and inferior to the contralateral greater trochanter.
- Manually lift and gather the soft tissue as the tape is applied to increase the stretch, and therefore tension, on the tape as the muscles contract into it.
- Lumbosacral strips should start slightly distal to the PSIS and run superiorly and medially to terminate the tension at L3/4. Note that the anchor point may extend above and below these points.
- This strip may be applied ipsilaterally and unilaterally if asymmetry is suspected, in order to resist counternutation and encourage low lumbar extension on that side; however, it is often performed bilaterally.

Re-evaluation
- Reassess the active straight-leg raise or other functional tasks that had demonstrated poor load-transfer capacity (e.g. single-leg standing, stairs).

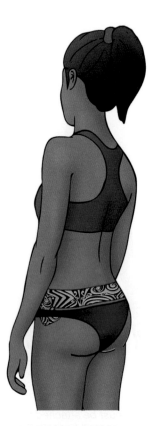

Figure 6.18: Dynamic taping for pelvic closure

Anterior Oblique Sling

Internal Obliques

Attachments

- Deep to external oblique
- Fibers emerge from lateral two-thirds of inguinal ligament, iliac crest, and TLF
- Posterior fibers pass almost vertically to invest into the tissues surrounding the inferior borders of the lower four ribs
- The anterior and lower fibers travel upward and medially, giving way to an aponeurosis (rectus sheath), and interlace with the linea alba
- The fibers arising from the inguinal ligament pass medially and downward, blending with the lower part of transversus abdominis and forming the conjoint tendon
- The conjoint tendon invests into the tissues surrounding the pubic crest and the pubis.

Innervation

- Lower six thoracic nerves (T7–T12)
- First lumbar nerve (L1).

Action

- Flexes trunk (concentric contraction of external oblique, internal oblique, and rectus abdominis bilaterally)
- If the ribs are fixed—lifts the anterior pelvis, altering the degree of pelvic tilt (decreasing lumbar lordosis)
- Rotation and lateral flexion of the trunk.

External Obliques

Attachments

- Located on the anterolateral aspect of the abdominal wall
- Fibers run downward and medially from the ribs toward the midline
- The upper attachment is to the outer borders of the lower eight ribs and their costal cartilages, interdigitating with serratus anterior above and latissimus dorsi below
- Fibers then run downward and medially, with those from the lower two ribs passing almost vertically to attach to the outer lip of the anterior two-thirds of the iliac crest, leaving a free posterior border of the muscle running between the twelfth rib and the iliac crest
- The remaining fibers give rise to a large aponeurosis that is broader below than above
- Each aponeurosis passes across rectus abdominis (rectus sheath), towards the midline to fuse with that from the opposite side at the linea alba (fibrous raphe running from the tip of the xiphoid process to the symphysis pubis)
- The lower, free border of the aponeurosis stretches between the pubic tubercle and the ASIS, forming the inguinal ligament.

Innervation

- By the anterior primary rami of nerves T7–T12
- Skin supplied by the same nerve roots.

Action

- Flexes trunk (concentric contraction of external oblique, internal oblique, and rectus abdominis bilaterally)
- If the ribs are fixed—lifts the anterior pelvis, altering the degree of pelvic tilt (decreasing lumbar lordosis)
- Rotation and lateral flexion of the trunk.

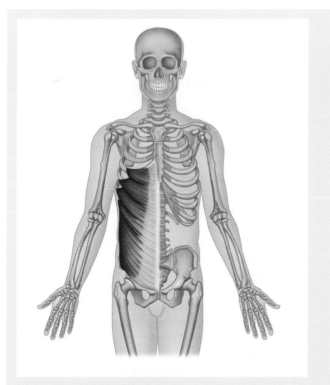

Figure 6.19: External oblique

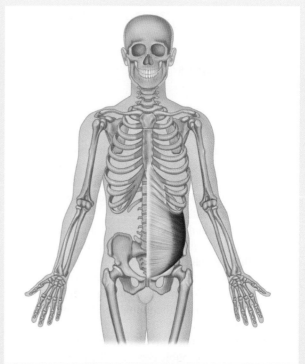

Figure 6.20: Internal oblique

Assessment for Strength

1. Athlete is supine, with hips and knees extended.
2. Stabilize athlete's pelvis and lower limbs.
3. Athlete attempts a diagonal sit up (arms by sides).
4. Offer resistance at the shoulder and contralateral hip.
5. Graded:
   - 5/5—strong contraction (normal)
   - 4/5—firm contraction (good)
   - 3/5—soft contraction (fair)
   - 2/5—slight contraction (poor)
   - 1/5—flicker (trace)
   - 0/5—no contraction detected.
6. Compare to the other side.
7. Reassess after treatment.

Soft-Tissue Treatment: Athlete Side-Lying

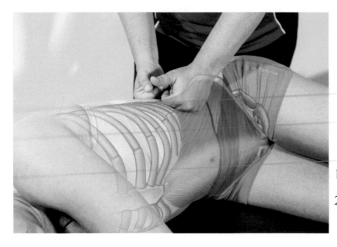

1. *Athlete is side-lying, with hips and knees slightly flexed for balance.*
2. *Sink the knuckles of both hands into the tissues just above the iliac crest (this can also be done with the ulnar border of your forearm).*

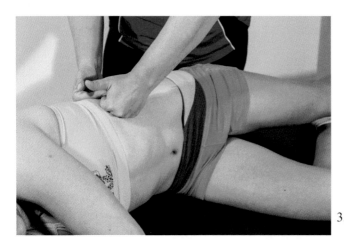

3. *Slowly direct the tissues proximally, lifting the tissues up and over the rib cage.*

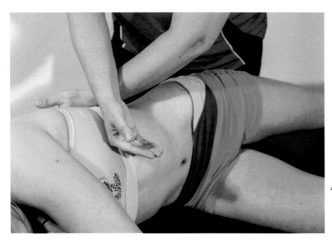

4. *When over the ribs, cross over hands with soft knuckles placed onto the skin and slowly open up the tissues by allowing the hands to move anteriorly and posteriorly over the ribs when the tissues allow.*

Adductor Magnus

Position and Attachments

- Largest and most posterior of the adductor group
- Adductor brevis and longus situated anteriorly
- Semimembranosus and semitendinosus situated posteriorly
- Composed of adductor and extensor fibers
- Upper fibers emerge from the femoral surface of the ischiopubic ramus
- Fibers travel downward to the lateral inferior surface of the ischial tuberosity
- Ischiopubic fibers fan out and form a large triangular sheet
  - *Anterior fibers pass laterally and slightly posteriorly to invest into the tissue surrounding the upper part of the linea aspera, then continue on to the greater trochanter*
  - *Fibers may be fused with quadratus femoris*
  - *Posterior fibers combine with the whole length of the linea aspera tissues and medial supracondylar ridge*
  - *Fibers pass downward and blend into the tissues surrounding the adductor tubercle*
  - *Some fibers fuse with the medial collateral ligament of the knee.*

Innervation

- Adductor part—posterior division of obturator nerve (root value L3, L3)
- Hamstring part—tibial division of sciatic nerve (root value L4)
- Skin covering inner thigh (L3).

Action

- As a whole—adduction of the hip joint
- Posterior portion aids in extension of the hip
- Together with adductor longus medially rotates the hip joint
- Prevention of lateral overbalancing during support phase of gait.

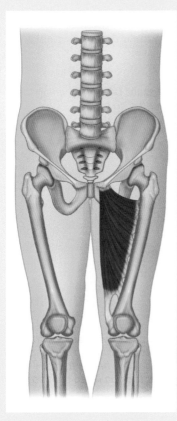

Figure 6.21: Adductor magnus

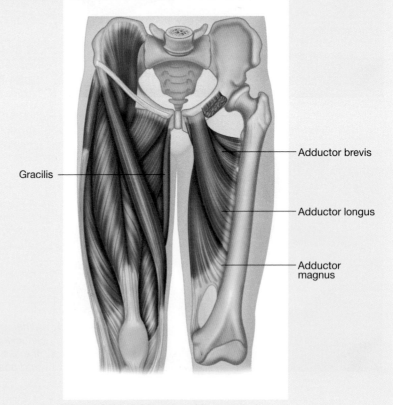

Gracilis

Adductor brevis

Adductor longus

Adductor magnus

Figure 6.22: Adductors with magnus in relation to brevis and longus

Palpation

1. This muscle is deep so can be difficult to palpate.
2. Athlete is side-lying with upper hip and knee flexed, resting on plinth.
3. Lower leg is extended.
4. Locate ischial tuberosity on the lower leg.
5. Athlete adducts hip; you will feel the strong band of adductor longus/gracilis.
6. Palpate posteriorly to this tendon and sink fingers in slowly until they have reached the tissues just superior to the medial condyle of the femur.
7. Athlete adducts to confirm location.

Assessment for Length

1. Athlete is supine, hips and knees flexed.
2. Hips externally rotated and plantar surface of feet facing each other.
3. Posterior pelvic tilt.
4. Athlete slowly lowers knees toward the plinth.
5. Does athlete anteriorly tilt the pelvis to hold the position?
   - Indicative of adductor shortness and abdominal weakness
   - Gluteus medius and hip external rotators may experience reciprocal inhibition, causing muscle imbalance and modified movement pattern.
6. Upper hip and thigh (possibly knee depending on flexibility) should be resting on plinth.
7. Reassess after treatment.

Assessment for Strength

1. Athlete is side-lying, with both legs extended.
2. Athlete abducts upper hip to approximately twenty-five degrees; hold athlete's leg at this position.
3. Athlete adducts the lower hip as you apply resistance.
   - Medial or lateral rotation of the hip is not permitted
   - Ipsilateral pelvic elevation is not permitted
   - Side flexion of the contralateral trunk is not permitted.
4. Stabilize athlete's pelvis and provide resistance proximal to the knee joint.
5. This is graded:
   - 5/5—strong contraction (normal)
   - 4/5—firm contraction (good)
   - 3/5—soft contraction (fair)
   - 2/5—slight contraction (poor)
   - 1/5—flicker (trace)
   - 0/5—no contraction detected.
6. Weakness may be due to inhibition, trigger points, pain, or muscle length.
7. Reassess after treatment.

For pectineus treatment, please see page 145.

Soft-Tissue Treatment: Athlete Supine 1

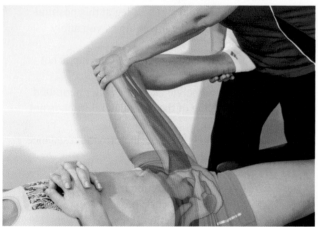

1. Stand on the side of the athlete to be treated.
2. Athlete has hip and knee flexed.
3. Place a towel between the athlete's legs for dignity.
4. Place athlete's foot on your thigh/hip and hold the ipsilateral knee.

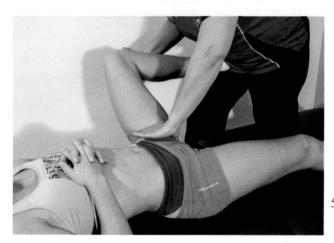

5. Sink into the tissues just distal to the ramus of the pubis and work along the length of the tissues distally.

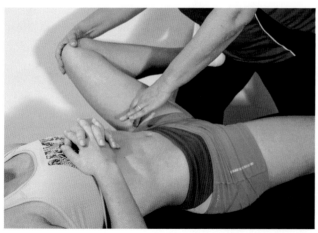

6. When the required depth has been reached, passively flex and externally rotate the ipsilateral hip by lunging forward.
7. Facilitate the movement by following with the contact hand (pressure maintained)—good for painful movements initially.
8. Resist the movement by locking into the tissues, maintaining that position whilst the tissues are actively or passively taken into position.

Soft-Tissue Treatment: Athlete Supine 2

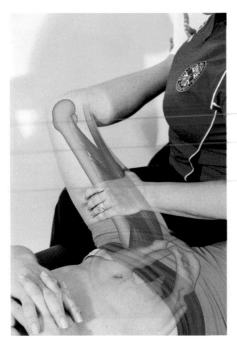

1. Passively abduct and externally rotate athlete's hip with knee flexed.

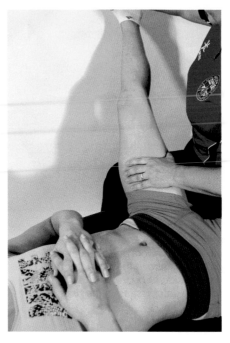

2. Contact the belly of the adductor magnus as above then passively extend the athlete's knee using the foot.

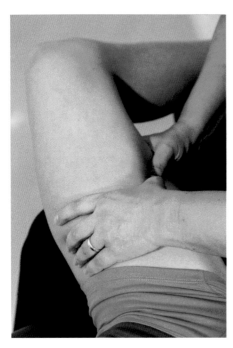

3. Sit or lean on the plinth with athlete's abducted and externally rotated hip resting on your thighs, then contact the belly of adductor magnus.

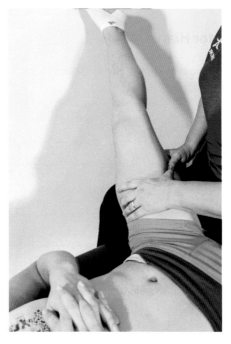

4. Athlete actively extends the knee.

Soft-Tissue Treatment: Athlete Side-Lying 1

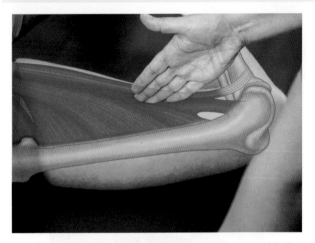

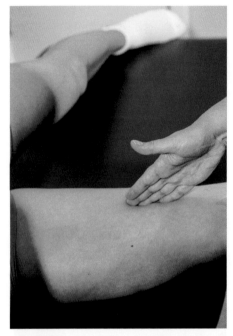

1. *Athlete has lower hip and knee flexed, upper hip in neutral, and upper knee extended.*
2. *Place all four fingers at approximately forty-five degrees, just above the adductor tubercle on the lower leg (side to be treated).*
3. *Sink slowly into tissues (remember VAS).*

4. *Direct tension proximally (cephalad direction); as tissues respond fingers will glide effortlessly—work between the tissue layers, focusing on areas that feel bound down.*
5. *Work delicately here—review your neurovascular anatomy (adductor hiatus).*
6. *Athlete slowly flexes and extends knee.*
7. *Repeat if necessary.*

Adductor Hiatus

Compression onto these delicate tissues is not advised.

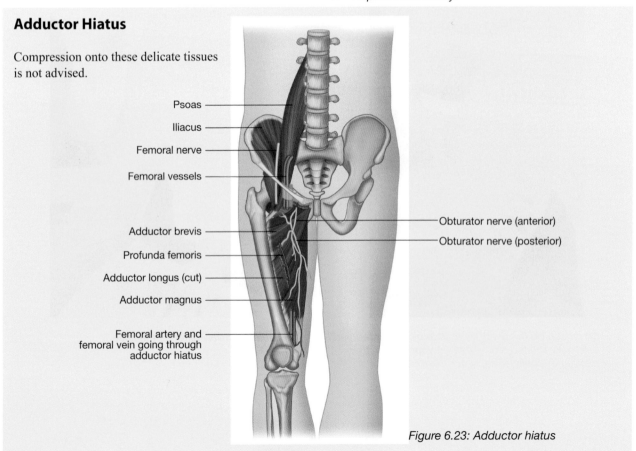

Psoas
Iliacus
Femoral nerve
Femoral vessels

Adductor brevis
Profunda femoris
Adductor longus (cut)
Adductor magnus

Femoral artery and femoral vein going through adductor hiatus

Obturator nerve (anterior)
Obturator nerve (posterior)

Figure 6.23: Adductor hiatus

Soft-Tissue Treatment: Athlete Side-Lying 2

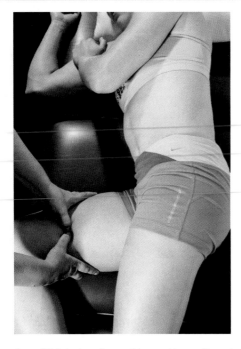 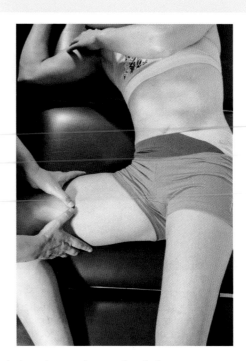

1. *Athlete has lower hip and knee flexed, upper hip in neutral, and upper knee extended.*
2. *Athlete's hips are perpendicular to the plinth.*
3. *Sink into tissues with soft thumbs above the adductor tubercle (remember to avoid the adductor hiatus) and maintain the depth (VAS).*
4. *Athlete rotates upper pelvis backward, controlling the discomfort (should never be above moderate discomfort).*

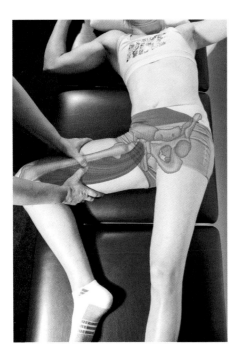

5. *As discomfort subsides, athlete rotates hip further and externally rotates the hip.*
   - *Athlete may need to place contralateral foot onto the plinth in order to fully rotate the pelvis*
6. *Is athlete able to complete this full external rotation?*
   - *Yes—athlete adds full horizontal abduction of contralateral arm*
   - *No—movement ends here as there will be too much stress on the tissues*
7. *Return to the starting position and repeat, working distally through the tissues.*

Soft-Tissue Treatment: Athlete Prone 1

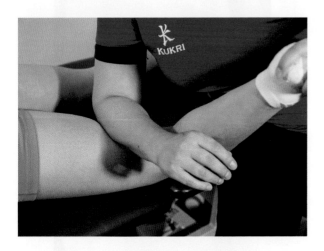 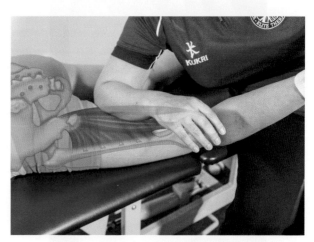

1. *Athlete is prone.*
2. *Stand on the side of the athlete to be treated.*
3. *Athlete's knee is passively flexed and hip medially rotated.*
4. *Using the ulnar border of the forearm, contact the belly of adductor magnus and slowly glide (tissue allowing) in a cephalad direction.*

Soft-Tissue Treatment: Athlete Prone 2

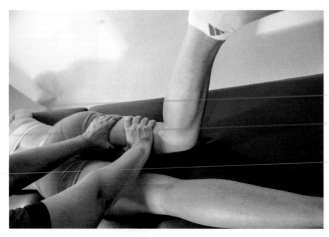

1. *Stand on the opposite side of the athlete to the one being treated.*
2. *Athlete flexes the knee on the side to be treated.*
3. *Sink your thumbs into the tissues of the adductor magnus (contact with the medial hamstrings will be inevitable) in the area between the pubis and the ischial tuberosity (VAS 6/10).*

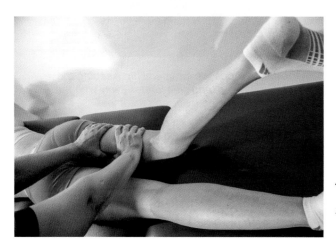

4. *Once the athlete is comfortable, the leg is slowly lowered (actively).*
5. *If increased discomfort is felt, the limb remains in this position until that discomfort subsides, the leg then continues to extend (VAS 2/10).*

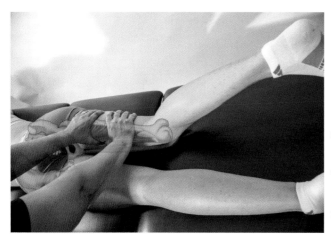

6. *Facilitate the movement by following with the contact hand (pressure maintained)—good for painful movements initially.*
7. *Resist the movement by locking into the tissues, maintaining that position whilst the tissues are actively or passively taken into position.*
8. *Continue this action until the entire length of the muscles has been addressed.*

Soft-Tissue Treatment: Athlete Standing

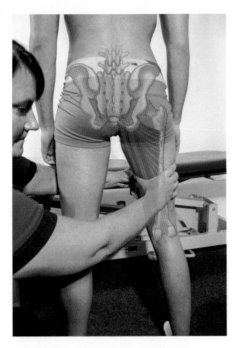

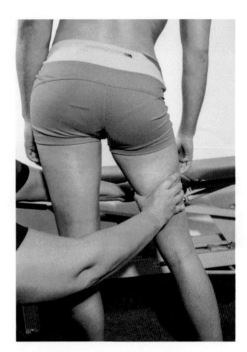

1. Athlete stands with feet just over hip width apart.
2. Kneel on the floor just behind the athlete's legs.
3. Contact the adductor group with soft thumbs or fingers below the pubis.

4. Athlete drops the ipsilateral hip (keeping the leg extended) and side lunges away with the contralateral leg by flexing the knee.

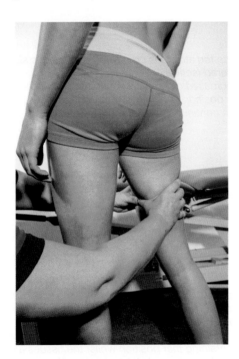

5. Athlete then rotates the trunk to the contralateral side (externally rotating the hip).
6. Work through the tissues, travelling distally.

Dry Needling for Adductors

Dry needling should only be performed by a qualified and insured physical therapist, owing to the invasive nature of the technique and serious anatomical considerations.

1. Note the referral pattern—does this represent your athlete's pain?
2. Athlete is supine, with hip and knee flexed, and hip externally rotated.
   - Avoid the sciatic nerve; femoral nerve, artery, and vein (see figure 6.36), and adductor canal.
3. Adductor longus and brevis:
   - Referral common to the knee

- Grasp muscle
- Longus—needle inserted anterior to posterior (A/P) into taut band/trigger point
- Brevis—needle between adductor longus and pectineus A/P.
4. Adductor magnus:
   - Referral common to anterior/medial thigh
   - Needle inserted perpendicularly, directly into taut band.
5. Gracilis:
   - Needle inserted perpendicularly, directly into taut band.

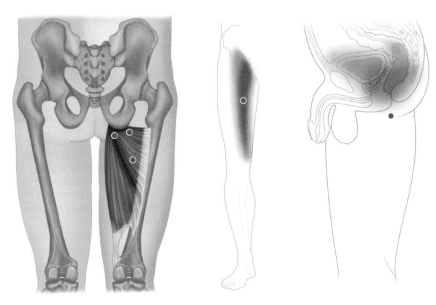

Figure 6.24: Adductor magnus trigger points and referral pattern

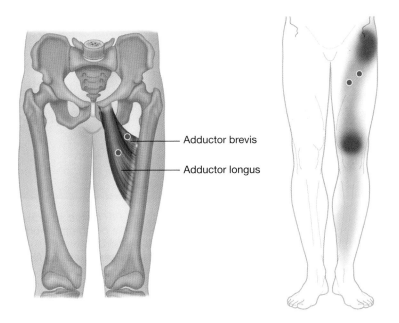

Adductor brevis

Adductor longus

Figure 6.25: Adductor longus and adductor brevis trigger points, and referral pattern

Instrument-Assisted Soft-Tissue Mobilization (IASTM): Athlete Standing

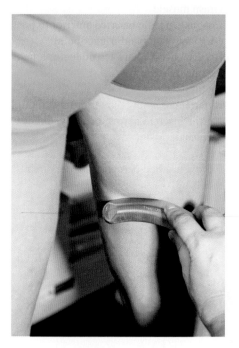 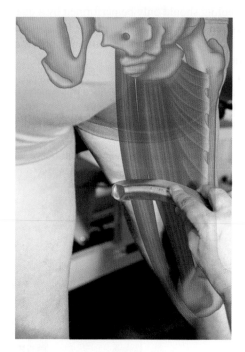

1. Athlete stands with feet just over hip width apart.
2. Kneel on the floor just behind the athlete's legs.
3. Use broad sweeping movements up and down and in an oblique direction (using the long curve).

4. Athlete simultaneously drops the ipsilateral hip (keeping the leg extended) and side lunges away with the contralateral leg by flexing the knee.
5. Athlete then rotates the trunk to the contralateral side (externally rotating the hip).
6. Repeat the broad sweeps, avoiding producing red bruising.

Muscle Energy Techniques (MET): Athlete Supine

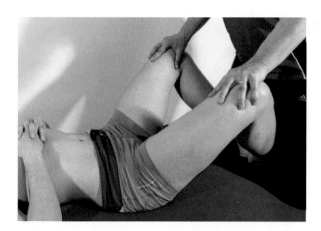 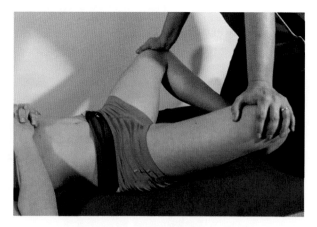

1. Athlete is supine, with hips and knees flexed and externally rotated, and plantar surfaces of the feet facing each other.
2. Gravity assists with this initial position, but open athlete's knees (hand contact on medial knees) into abduction/external rotation until resistance is felt (starting point).
3. Athlete adducts hips against your resistance, using approximately twenty percent of overall strength for ten to twelve seconds.

4. Utilizing the PIR period (approximately twenty seconds), take both femurs further into abduction/external rotation.
5. Repeat these steps until no further gains are achieved.

Additional Structures Impacting on SIJ Function

Quadratus Lumborum

Attachments

- Invests into the tissues surrounding the iliolumbar ligament and the adjacent posterior surface of the iliac crest
- Fibers run upward and medially to invest into the tissues surrounding the lateral anterior surface of the transverse processes L1–L5 and the medial lower border of the twelfth rib
- Enclosed within the anterior and middle layers of the TLF.

Innervation

- Anterior primary rami of the subcostal nerve and upper three or four lumbar nerves (root value T12, L1–L4).

Action

- Lateral flexion of the trunk to the ipsilateral side
- Standing on one leg—prevents the pelvis from dropping downward on the contralateral side
- Steadies twelfth rib during deep inspiration (fixed diaphragm)
- Bilateral action helps lumbar extension and gives lateral stability.

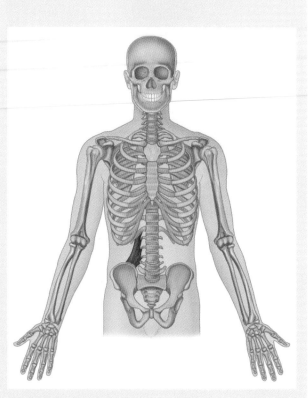

Figure 6.26: Quadratus lumborum (QL)

Palpation

1. Athlete is prone.
2. Locate twelfth rib, transverse processes of lumbar vertebrae, and posterior iliac crest.
3. The tissues of the QL lie between these points.
4. Visualize the tissues, and sink slowly but firmly through the lumbar fascia toward the vertebrae.
5. Athlete can hitch his or her pelvis (upward lateral tilt) to initiate a contraction and confirm location.

Soft-Tissue Treatment: Athlete Prone 1

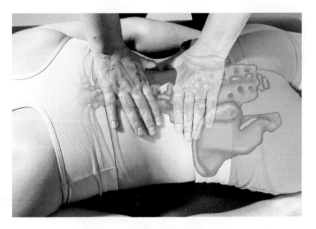

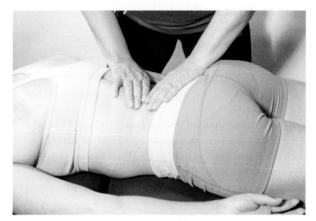

1. *Using your thumb pads, slowly melt into the tissues distal to the twelfth rib and lateral to the QL.*
2. *Sink in further by travelling medially toward the vertebrae (again using VAS).*

3. *Once the athlete is comfortable with this depth, the hip is pulled downward (downward tilt) slowly.*
   - *Facilitate the movement by following the downward direction of the tissues with the contact thumbs (pressure maintained)—good for painful movements initially.*
   - *Resist the movement by locking into the tissues, maintaining that position whilst the tissues are actively taken into position.*
4. *Repeat this sequence, working carefully from the twelfth rib to edge of the ilium.*

Soft-Tissue Treatment: Athlete Prone 1 (if another person is available)

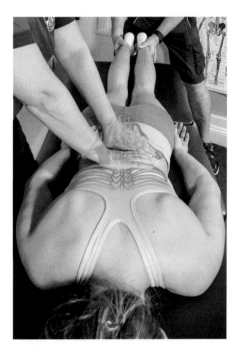

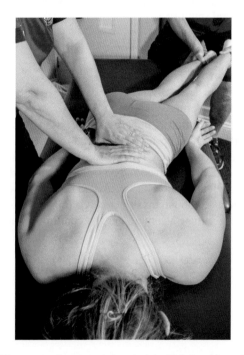

1. *Follow the directions above (points 1–3).*

2. *The second person takes hold of bilateral legs (just above the ankles) and slowly takes the ipsilateral leg into adduction and the contralateral leg into abduction (moving both legs at the same time).*

Soft-Tissue Treatment: Side-Lying 1

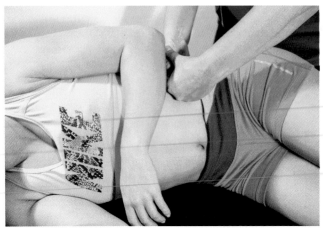

1. Place a cushion or bolster between the athlete's knees.
2. Athlete's upper elbow is flexed and arm adducted.
3. Contact the lateral tissues on the edge of the ilium with soft knuckles or forearm.
4. Slowly melt into the tissues (VAS) and sweep upward (very slowly) toward the ribs.

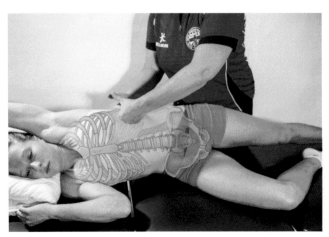

5. Initially adding shoulder abduction and leg extension would cause the fascia to tighten over the ribs, but after a few sweeps adding shoulder abduction is effective if performed slowly.

Soft-Tissue Treatment: Side-Lying 2

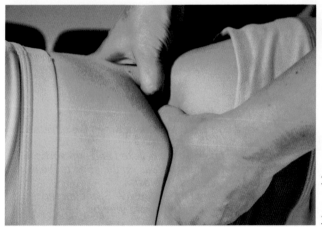

1. *Athlete's hips and knees are flexed, and arm is relaxed as above.*
2. *Face cephalad and sink your thumb pads into the lateral tissues (one hand resting over the abdomen and one hand resting over the lumbar tissues).*
3. *Maintain pressure.*

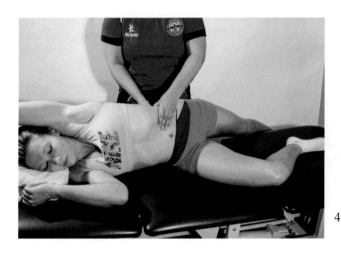

4. *Athlete actively extends hip and flexes shoulder slowly...*

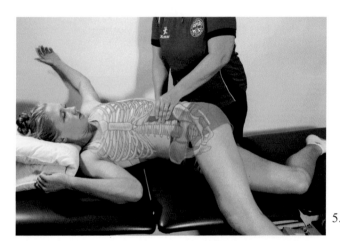

5. *...followed by hip flexion and adduction with shoulder horizontal abduction.*

Soft-Tissue Treatment: Athlete Standing

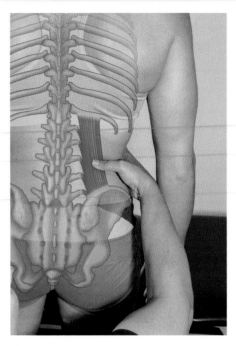

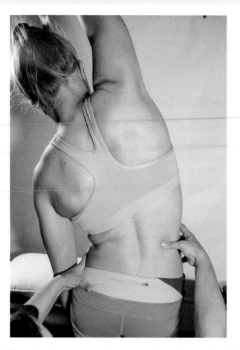

1. *Athlete stands in neutral.*
2. *Engage the lateral tissues with flat fingertips or thumb.*

3. *Athlete begins to reach upward and into side flexion as the tissues are taken in the same direction.*

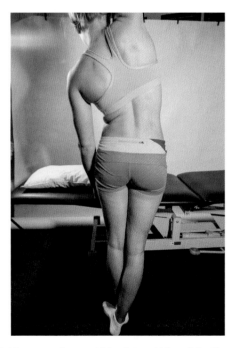

4. *Athlete can then add ipsilateral hip adduction, crossing that leg behind the other.*

The Fascial Relationship of QL with the Iliacus

Follow the step-by-step instructions for the iliacus shown later in this chapter—owing to the fascial relationship (see Figure 6.27), working in this area is imperative as it helps reduce QL hypertonicity.

Dry Needling for Quadratus Lumborum

Dry needling should only be performed by a qualified and insured physical therapist, owing to the invasive nature of the technique and serious anatomical considerations.

1. Athlete is prone/supine/side-lying.
2. Note referral pattern—does this represent your athlete's pain?
3. Referral is generally deep and aching.
4. Commonly referring to the groin and SIJ (medial trigger points).
5. When athlete is side-lying, locate by following palpation instructions above.
6. Use a long needle (it needs to travel through latissimus dorsi if above L4).
7. Needle directly toward the transverse processes.
8. Avoid penetrating the kidney, diaphragm, and pleura (needle below L2).

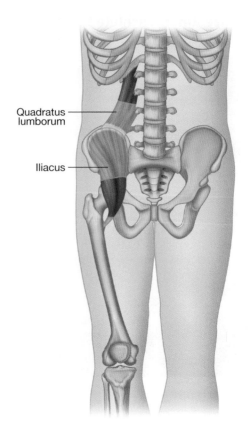

Figure 6.27: The fascial relationship of QL with the iliacus

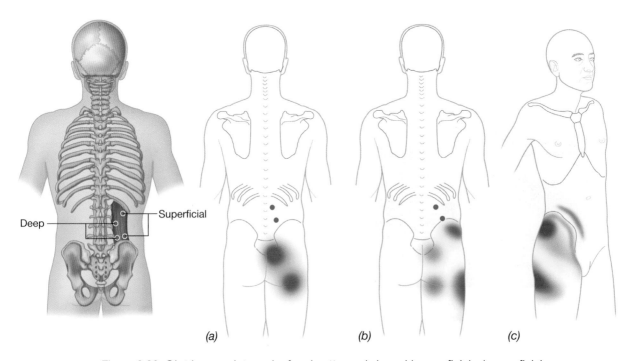

Figure 6.28: QL trigger points and referral pattern, a) deep, b) superficial, c) superficial

Muscle Energy Techniques (MET): Athlete Side-Lying

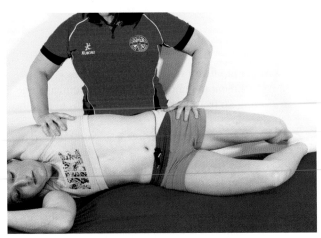

1. *Lower leg is flexed at the hip and knee.*
2. *Upper leg is adducted over the edge of the plinth.*
3. *Upper arm is holding onto the top of the plinth.*
4. *Stabilize athlete's thorax with one hand and contact the femur just above the knee with the other.*
5. *Athlete abducts femur using approximately twenty percent of their overall strength for ten to twelve seconds.*
6. *Utilizing the PIR period (approximately twenty seconds), take the femur into further adduction (maintaining thorax position with the other hand).*
7. *Repeat these steps until no further gains are achieved.*

Muscle Energy Techniques (MET): Alternative

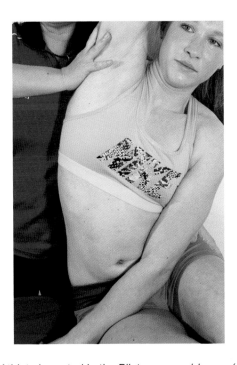

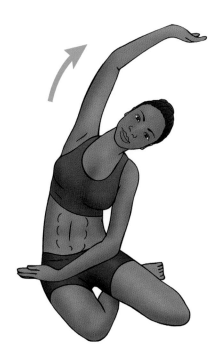

1. *Athlete is seated in the Pilates mermaid pose (see illustration).*
2. *Repeat the steps above, this time resisting the side flexion of the thorax.*

Psoas Major

Attachments and Location

- Within its substance is the lumbar plexus
- At its upper end, the diaphragm and medial arcuate ligament lie anteriorly
- Its right side is overlapped by the inferior vena cava and the ileum
- The upper fibers invest into the adjacent margins of the bodies of vertebrae T12–L5 and the discs in between, as well as the anterior and medial parts of each transverse process
- Fibers pass downward and forward toward the pelvis (where they connect with those of the iliacus), under the inguinal ligament
- Fibers become more vertical at this point, then pass downward and backward laterally
- It is separated from the pubis and hip joint capsule by a large bursa
- Its fibers invest into the tissue surrounding the posterior aspect of the lesser trochanter of the femur.

Innervation

- Anterior rami of L1–L3 (sometimes L4)
- Small area of skin (groin area) L1.

Action

- Major hip flexor of the hip joint
- Attachment to lumbar spine—flexes lumbar spine
- Sitting up from lying—bilaterally helps to pull the trunk up
  - Abdominal muscles are also working hard to flex the trunk
  - Important that they are working well as this will prevent the lumbar spine being drawn forward before the trunk begins to rise
  - Pulling the head up first will prevent this un-wanted/potentially damaging movement from occurring
- Giving clarity as to why raising both limbs at the same time in the supine position can lead to back pain.

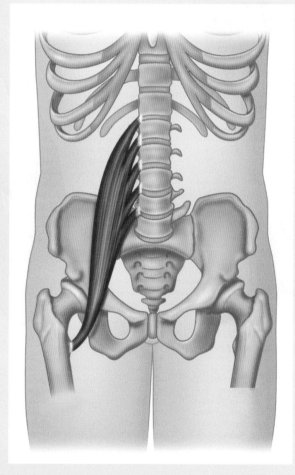

Figure 6.29: Psoas major

Inhibition of the Psoas

Owing to the reciprocal relationship between the GM and the psoas (where one may inhibit the other), assessing to determine whether the psoas is inhibited gives important information. This can be done in the supine position with the hip flexed (knee extended) and slightly laterally rotated (picture shows a common compensatory hand position the athlete will adopt, when testing ensure athlete's hands are by their sides). One hand stabilizes the contralateral pelvis while the other pushes the ipsilateral leg toward the plinth (as the athlete attempts to maintain the initial position). Inhibition is indicated if the leg is pushed onto the table with ease or if there are compensatory movements from the neck, feet, torso, shoulders, or arms.

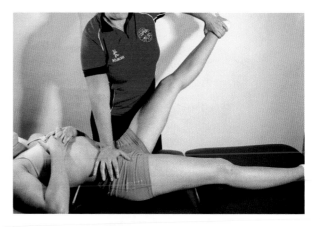

Figure 6.30. Activation process

1. Athlete should be able to hold the position against resistance.
2. If not, this does not necessarily indicate weakness (in most cases with athletes it definitely does not) but is more likely to be inhibited.
3. Athlete should perform supine diaphragmatic breathing prior to training until he or she is able to perform this sitting and standing without effort (Figure 6.33).

The Diaphragm

The diaphragm has multiple origins—from the inner surfaces of ribs seven to twelve, medial surfaces of vertebral bodies L1–L3, the anterior longitudinal ligament, the posterior surface of the xiphoid process, and the arcuate ligament, connecting to the aorta, psoas, and the QL to insert into the central tendon.

The medial arcuate ligament is a continuation of the superior psoas fascia that continues superiorly to the diaphragm. The right and left crura make up the spinal attachment of the diaphragm. They attach to the anterolateral components of the upper three lumbar vertebrae and their bodies. The crura and their fascia overlap psoas and appear continuous with psoas until they come more anteriorly and blend with the anterior longitudinal ligament (Gibbons, 2001). As psoas descends, its inferomedial fascia becomes thick at its lower portion and is continuous with the pelvic floor fascia. This also forms a link with the conjoint tendon, transversus abdominis, and the internal oblique.

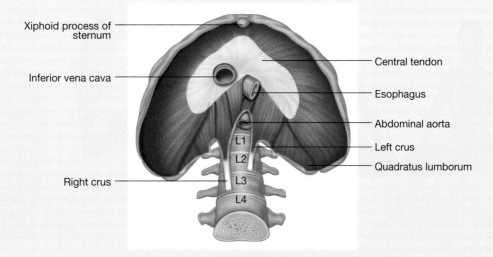

Figure 6.31. Demonstrating the multiple origins of the diaphragm

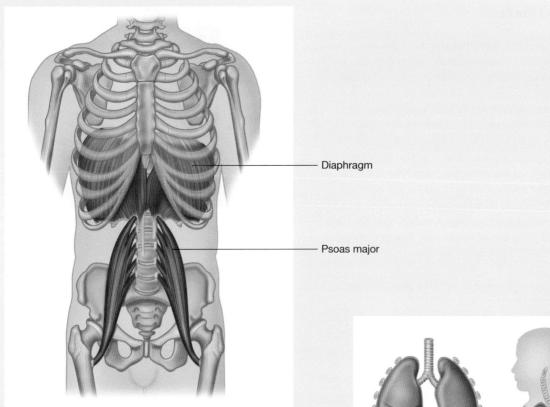

Figure 6.32. Demonstrating the intimate relationship between the diaphragm and the psoas

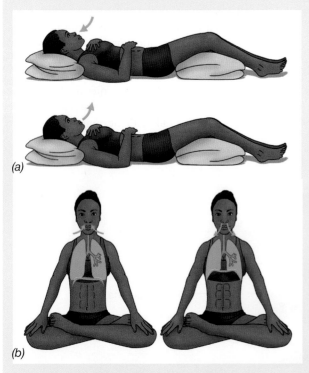

Figure 6.33: Diaphragmatic motion is greater in the supine position (a) than in the erect or sitting position (b) because the postural control exercised by the crural portion of the diaphragm is eliminated in the supine position, allowing greater excursion (Takazakura et al., 2004)

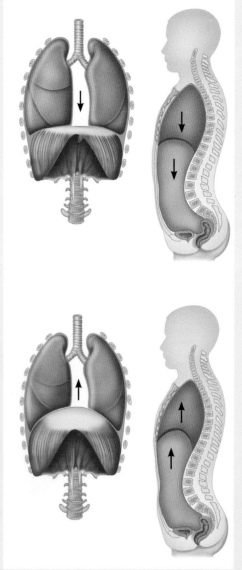

Figure 6.34. Diaphragmatic breathing

Palpation

1. Athlete is supine—crook lying.
2. Locate the belly button and the ASIS.
3. With soft finger pads, very slowly sink your fingers between these two points (slightly medially toward the spine), allowing the abdominal aponeurosis to soften and the abdominal contents to move aside.
4. The psoas lies very close to the abdominal aorta, so this palpation must be slow; at any time a pulse is detected, fingers must be angled away.
5. Athlete inhales deeply and, on exhalation, sink your fingers in further.
6. Athlete can flex the hip to initiate a contraction and confirm location.

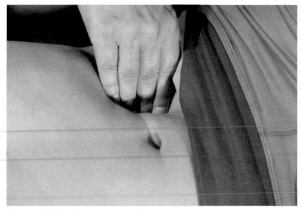

Figure 6.35: Psoas palpation

Assessment for Length

Modified Thomas Test

1. Athlete is seated on the end of the plinth.
2. Athlete flexes one hip and knee; help athlete to lie back onto the plinth.
3. Athlete completely relaxes the extended leg.
   - Lumbar extension is not permitted.
   - Does the thigh rest on the plinth?
     - *Yes and thigh is in neutral = normal*
     - *Yes but thigh is laterally rotated = short sartorius*
     - *Yes but the knee is extended = short rectus femoris*
     - *Yes but the hip is medially rotated/ abducted = short tensor fascia latae*
     - *Yes but the hip is adducted = short pectineus or adductor longus*
     - *No = short iliopsoas, adductor longus, and pectineus*
4. Reassess after treatment.

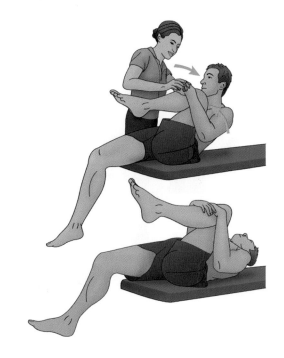

Figure 6.36: Modified Thomas test

Assessment for Strength

1. Athlete is seated.
2. Athlete flexes hip and knee above ninety degrees.
3. Stabilize athlete's contralateral pelvis.
4. Athlete flexes hip against your resistance (proximal to knee joint).
5. Graded:
   - 5/5—strong contraction (normal)
   - 4/5—firm contraction (good)
   - 3/5—soft contraction (fair)
   - 2/5—slight contraction (poor)
   - 1/5—flicker (trace)
   - 0/5—no contraction detected.
6. Weakness may be due to inhibition, trigger points, pain, or muscle length.
7. Reassess after treatment.

Soft-Tissue Treatment: Athlete Supine 1

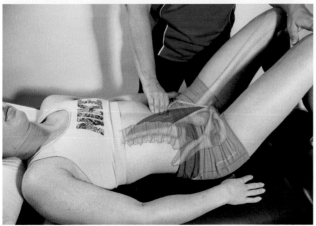

1. Athlete is in crook-lying position.
2. Palpate the psoas as above.
3. Whilst you maintain pressure, athlete flexes both arms to ninety degrees.

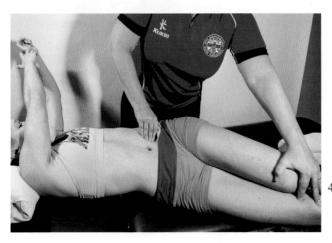

4. Whilst you maintain pressure, athlete slowly rolls the knees ipsilaterally as the arms horizontally abduct and adduct to the contralateral side (move both arms at the same time).

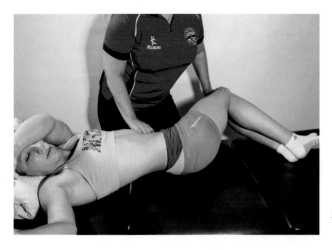

5. This is immediately followed by the exact opposite movement of the knees and the arms.

Soft-Tissue Treatment: Athlete Supine 2

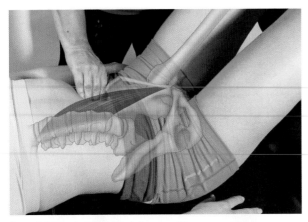

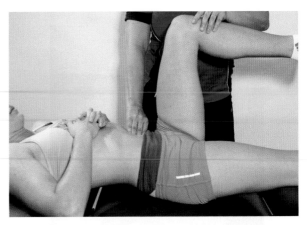

1. Athlete is in crook-lying position.
2. Palpate the psoas as above.
3. Whilst you maintain pressure, athlete slowly tilts the pelvis anteriorly and posteriorly, two or three times.

4. Whilst you maintain pressure, athlete flexes the ipsilateral hip (knee flexed).

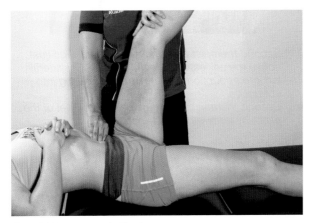

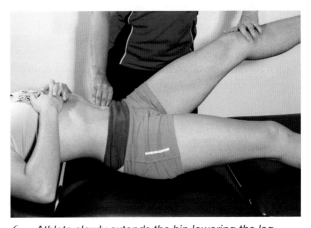

5. Athlete extends the knee.

6. Athlete slowly extends the hip lowering the leg toward the plinth.

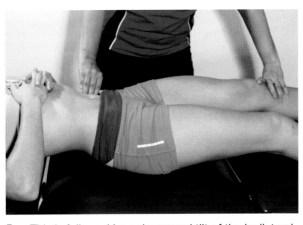

7. This is followed by a downward tilt of the ipsilateral pelvis.
8. Facilitate the movement by following the downward direction of the tissues with the contact fingers (pressure maintained)—good for painful movements initially.

Soft-Tissue Treatment: Athlete Supine 3 (if another person is available)

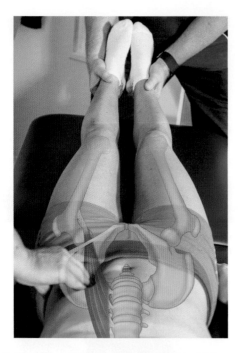
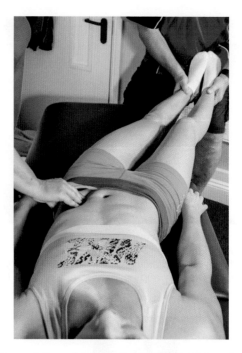

1. Follow the palpation directions (page 135).
2. First therapist maintains pressure on tissues above the psoas.

3. Second therapist takes hold of bilateral legs (just above the ankles) and slowly takes the ipsilateral leg into adduction and the contralateral leg into abduction.
4. Second therapist takes legs below the level of the plinth by adding bilateral knee flexion.

Soft-Tissue Treatment: Athlete Side-Lying

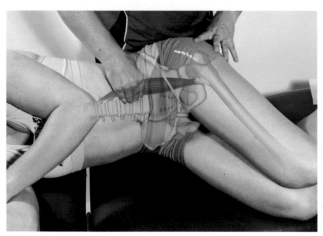

1. This is a good position for anyone with increased abdominal adipose tissue as gravity allows these tissues and the abdominal tissues (mesentery) to move away from the psoas.
2. Athlete has hips and knees flexed, and a pillow or bolster between the knees.
3. Locate the psoas as before, this time sliding down the iliacus (same speed and care must be taken).
4. Whilst you maintain the pressure, the athlete slowly extends and medially rotates the ipsilateral hip.

Dry Needling for Psoas Major

Dry needling of the psoas (I only ever needle the lower trigger point) should only be performed by a qualified and insured physical therapist, owing to the invasive nature of the technique and serious anatomical considerations.

1. Note the referral pattern—does this represent your athlete's pain?
2. Athlete is supine.
3. Athlete's hip is flexed, externally rotated, and supported by a pillow.
4. Avoid the femoral artery in the femoral triangle (see Figure 6.37; check pulse).
5. Needle the lower trigger point by ensuring you are approximately one finger's breadth lateral to the femoral artery, then needle in a lateral direction.

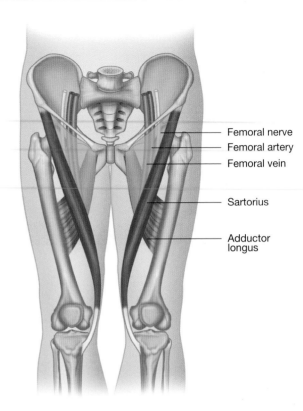

Femoral nerve
Femoral artery
Femoral vein

Sartorius

Adductor longus

Figure 6.37: Femoral triangle

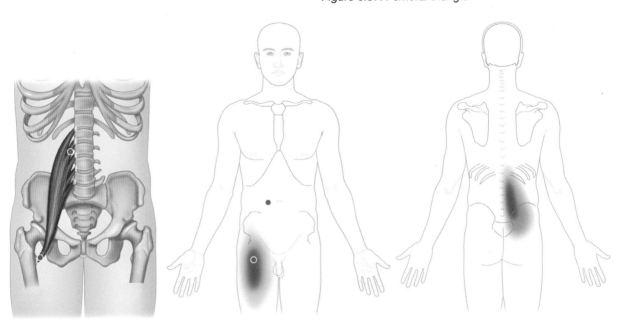

Figure 6.38: Psoas trigger points and referral pattern

Muscle Energy Techniques (MET) (Psoas and Iliacus): Athlete Supine

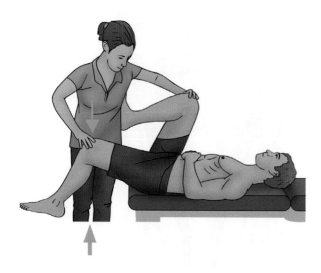

1. Athlete adopts the modified Thomas test position (see Figure 6.36).
2. Assess the hip for hypertonicity:
   - Psoas—femur higher than hip joint, not resting on plinth
   - Tensor fascia latae (TFL)/iliotibial tract (ITT)—hip abducted
   - Adductors—hip adducted
   - Quadriceps femoris—knee extended
   - Or combinations of the above.
3. For psoas hypertonicity/shortness, the modified Thomas test position is the starting point.
4. Gravity helps determine where the resistance of the tissues begins, but this resistance should also be determined by taking the hip into extension passively, until resistance is felt.
5. Athlete flexes hip/femur using approximately twenty percent of overall strength for ten to twelve seconds.
6. Utilizing the PIR period (approximately twenty seconds), take the femur into extension (maintaining pelvic position with the other hand).
7. Repeat these steps until no further gains are achieved.

Iliacus

Attachments

- Upper posterior two-thirds of the tissue surrounding the iliac fossa
- Some fibers come from the ala of the sacrum and anterior sacroiliac ligament
- Fibers pass downward, forward and medially, blending with the lateral side of psoas major.

Innervation

- Femoral nerve root (root value L2 and L3)
- Skin covering (L1).

Action

- If the upper attachment is fixed—pulls thigh forward as in flexion of the hip
- Lower attachment fixed—draws pelvis forward (tilting)
- Functional activity same as psoas major.

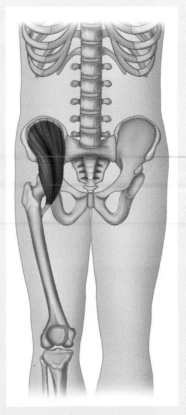

Figure 6.39: Iliacus

Palpation

1. Athlete is supine—crook lying.
2. Side to be palpated is laterally rotated and supported on your thigh.
3. Locate the iliac crest.
4. Athlete inhales; on exhalation slowly sink your curled fingers toward the iliac fossa.
5. Athlete can flex the hip to initiate a contraction and confirm location.

Soft-Tissue Treatment: Athlete Supine 1

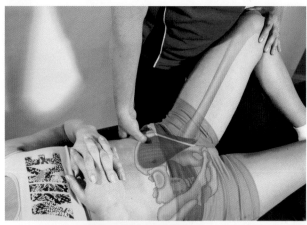

1. *Palpate the tissues as directed above.*
2. *Whilst you maintain pressure, the athlete adducts the ipsilateral knee against your resistance.*

3. *Then push the knee into adduction, taking advantage of the PIR.*

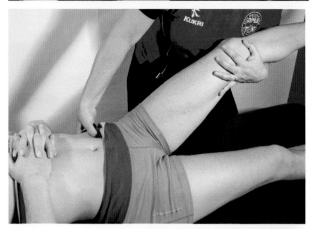

4. *Then take it immediately into external rotation, hip and knee extension (hook arm under athlete's knee), and pull it into distraction.*
5. *Repeat this action after moving contact fingers distally/deeper into the iliacus tissues.*

Soft-Tissue Treatment: Athlete Supine 2

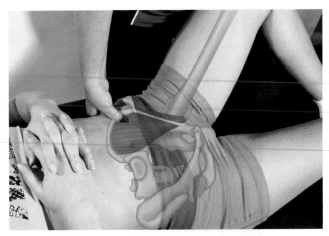

1. Athlete is positioned as above.
2. Whilst you maintain pressure, the athlete slowly tilts the pelvis anteriorly and posteriorly two or three times.
3. Whilst you maintain pressure, the athlete performs a very small bridging movement.
   - Facilitate the movement by following the downward direction of the tissues with the contact fingers (pressure maintained)—good for painful movements initially.
   - Resist the movement by locking into the tissues, maintaining that position whilst the tissues are actively taken into position.
4. Return the pelvis to neutral.
5. Whilst you maintain pressure, the athlete performs a downward tilt of the pelvis.

Soft-Tissue Treatment: Athlete Side-Lying

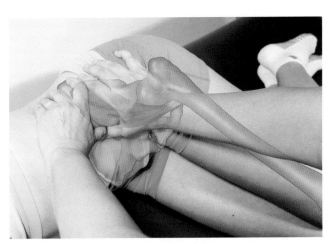

1. Athlete has hips and knees flexed, with pillow/bolster between the knees.
2. Palpate the tissues surrounding the iliacus as before.

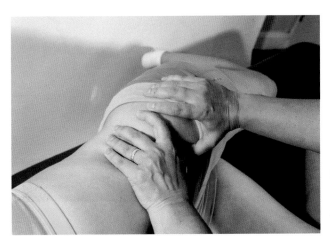

3. Alternatively, turn and face the athlete and palpate the tissues using both thumb pads (slowly and gently as before).
4. Whilst you maintain pressure, the athlete slowly extends the hip.

Soft-Tissue Treatment: Athlete Standing

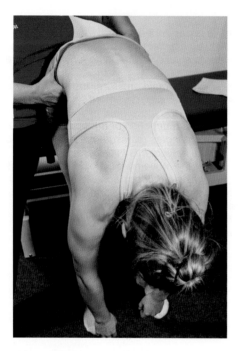

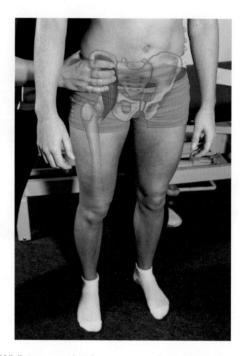

1. *Athlete adopts lumbar flexion.*
2. *Engage tissues as before.*

3. *Whilst you maintain pressure, the athlete returns to neutral slowly.*

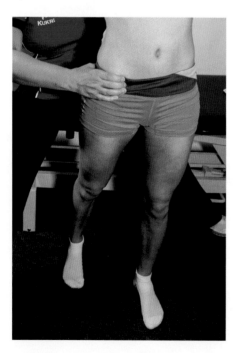

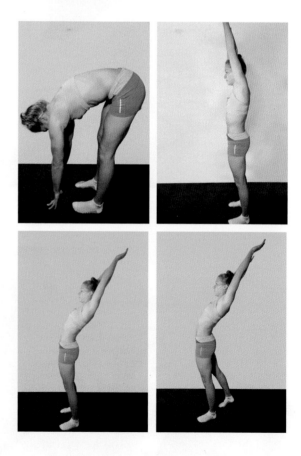

4. *Athlete then adds lumbar and thoracic extension.*
5. *This can be followed by ipsilateral hip extension.*
6. *This is a strong technique and not for the faint hearted.*

Dry Needling for Iliacus

Dry needling should only be performed by a qualified and insured physical therapist, owing to the invasive nature of the technique and serious anatomical considerations.

1. Note the referral pattern—does this represent your athlete's pain?
2. Athlete is supine.
3. Athlete's hip is flexed, externally rotated, and supported by a pillow.
4. Palpate the area of soft tissue adjacent to ASIS.
5. Direct the needle posteriorly toward the iliac fossa.
6. Care must be taken to not pierce the sciatic and femoral neurovascular structures.

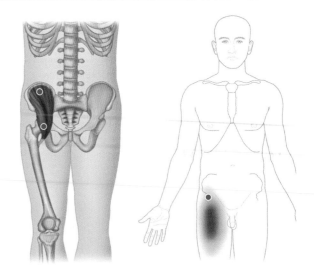

Figure 6.40: Iliacus trigger points and referral pattern

Pectineus

Pectineus has been included here rather than with the adductors owing to its intimate relationship with the psoas and pelvic position.

Attachments

- Upper fibers invest into the superior ramus of the pubis, the iliopubic eminence and the pubic tubercle
- Fibers also invest into the fascia that covers pectineus
- Fibers pass downward, backward, and laterally between psoas major and the adductor longus
- Fibers invest in the tissues surrounding the lesser trochanter and the linea aspera of the femur.

Innervation

- Femoral nerve (root value L2 and L3)
- Occasionally obturator or accessory obturator nerve (root value L3)
- Skin covering (L1).

Action

- Flexes and adducts the hip joint
- Draws the thigh inward and forward (rotational element not confirmed).

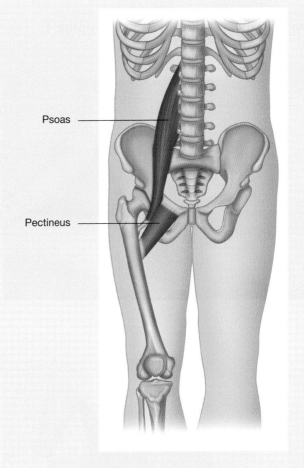

Figure 6.41: Pectineus

Palpation

1. Athlete is supine.
2. Athlete's hip is flexed and externally rotated, resting on your thigh.
3. Locate the tendon of adductor longus or gracilis by asking the athlete to adduct against resistance.
4. Move fingers laterally away from the tendon and sink slowly into the tissues of the pectineus.
5. Athlete can flex the hip, aiming for the contralateral shoulder, to initiate a contraction and confirm location. Alternatively, active adduction will confirm location.

Soft-Tissue Treatment: Athlete Supine 1

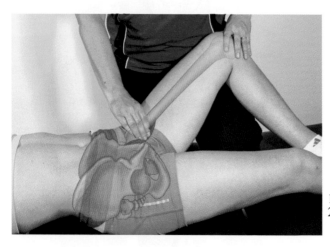

1. *Athlete is supine.*
2. *Locate the tissues of pectineus as in Palpation, above.*

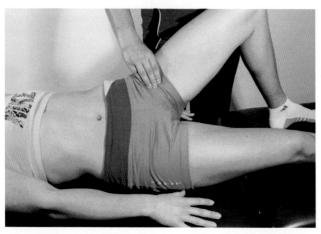

3. *Whilst you maintain pressure, the athlete places the ipsilateral foot onto the plinth. Athlete then pushes into the plinth with the foot and lifts the ipsilateral hip, rotating it toward the contralateral side.*
   - *Facilitate the movement by following the downward direction of the tissues with the contact fingers (pressure maintained)—good for painful movements initially.*
   - *Resist the movement by locking into the tissues, maintaining that position whilst the tissues are actively taken into position.*

Soft-Tissue Treatment: Athlete Supine 2

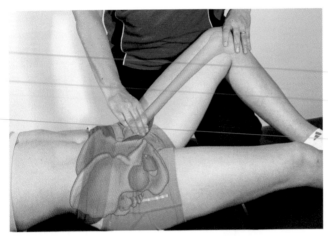

1. *Athlete is supine.*
2. *Face the athlete in a caudad direction.*
3. *Locate the tissues of pectineus as in Palpation, page 146.*

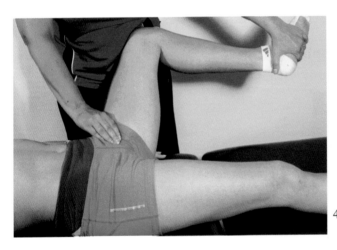

4. *Maintaining pressure, grasp the athlete's ipsilateral foot and take the hip into flexion and abduction.*

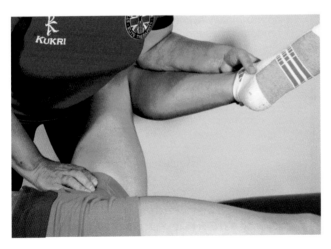

5. *Contact the medial aspect of the ipsilateral knee with your forearm (and the hand holding the athlete's foot), and block this position while adding external rotation of the hip, by lifting the foot toward the ceiling.*

Dry Needling for Pectineus

Dry needling should only be performed by a qualified and insured physical therapist, owing to the invasive nature of the technique and serious anatomical considerations.

1. Note the referral pattern—does this represent your athlete's pain?
2. Athlete is supine, positioned as above.
3. Palpation of the femoral artery is important (see page 139); once you locate it, keep one finger in place.
4. Palpate tissues for taut band.
5. Insert the needle perpendicularly to the muscle and medially to the femoral artery.
6. Avoid needling any of the delicate structures in the femoral triangle and the obturator nerve (close to adductor longus attachment, see page 114).

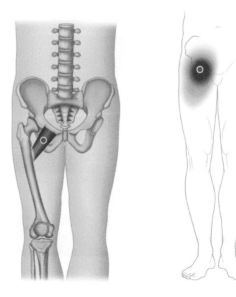

Figure 6.42: Pectineus trigger points and referral pattern

Muscle Energy Techniques (MET): Athlete Supine

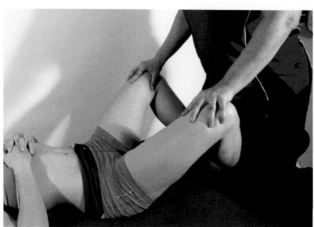

1. Athlete is supine.
2. Athlete's hips and knees are flexed and externally rotated, with the plantar surfaces of the feet facing each other.
3. Gravity assists with this initial position, but you should open both knees (hand contact on medial knees) into abduction/external rotation until you feel resistance (starting point).
4. Athlete adducts hips against your resistance using approximately twenty percent of overall strength for ten to twelve seconds.

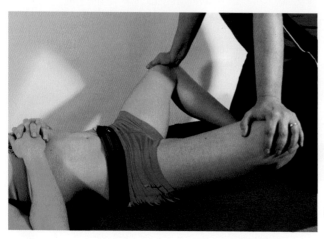

5. Utilizing the PIR period (approximately twenty seconds), take both femurs further into abduction/external rotation.
6. Repeat these steps until no further gains are achieved.

Tensor Fascia Latae

Attachments

- Fibers invest into the tissues surrounding the anterior part of the outer lip of iliac crest:
  - Between and including the iliac tubercle and the anterior superior iliac spine
  - The area of the gluteal surface just below that
  - The fascia between the muscle and the gluteus minimus, and that covering its surface
- Fibers inferiorly invest into the tissues between the two layers of the iliotibial tract (ITT), below the level of the greater trochanter.

Innervation

- Superior gluteal nerve (root value L4 and L5)
- Skin covering (L1).

Action

- Overlies gluteus minimus and helps flex, abduct, and medially rotate the hip joint
- Acting with superficial fibers of GM it tightens the ITT and extends the knee joint (distal fibers invest into lateral condyle of tibia)
- Acting with gluteus minimus it medially rotates the hip joint
- Posterior fibers may help in abduction of the thigh
- Helps control the movements of the pelvis and femur on the tibia in weight bearing
- Strong medial rotator when the hip is in extension and the lower limb, pelvis, and trunk are prepared following the "toe-off" phase of walking
- Inhibition of the quadriceps can lead to the overdevelopment of the TFL.

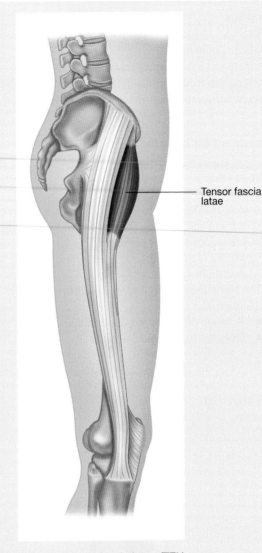

Tensor fascia latae

Figure 6.43. Tensor fascia latae (TFL)

Palpation

1. Athlete is supine.
2. Palpate just posterior and distal to ASIS.
3. Athlete can medially rotate the hip, aiming to initiate a contraction and confirm location.

Assessment for Length

Modified Ober's Test

1. Athlete is side-lying.
2. Lower hip and knee are slightly flexed for stability and to reduce anterior pelvic tilt.
3. Upper leg is extended.
4. Abduct and hyperextend the hip.
5. The hip is then slowly lowered (adducting toward the plinth).
   - Rotation of the hip is not permitted.
   - Does the thigh remain abducted?
     - *Yes = short TFL.*
     - *No, the hip adducts and rests on the table = TFL normal.*
6. Reassess after treatment.

Assessment for Strength

1. Athlete is side-lying.
2. Lower leg is extended.
3. Upper hip is flexed to forty-five degrees, with knee extended and limb resting on the plinth.
4. Athlete abducts hip, maintaining forty-five degrees of flexion.
5. Stabilize athlete's pelvis.
6. Resist by applying pressure proximal to knee joint.
7. This is graded:
   - 5/5—strong contraction (normal)
   - 4/5—firm contraction (good)
   - 3/5—soft contraction (fair)
   - 2/5—slight contraction (poor)
   - 1/5—flicker (trace)
   - 0/5—no contraction detected.
8. Weakness may be due to inhibition, trigger points, pain, or muscle length.
9. Reassess after treatment.

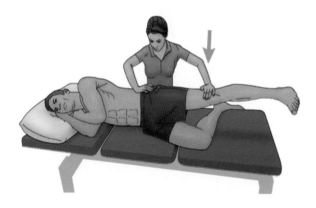

Figure 6.44: Modified Ober's test

Soft-Tissue Treatment: Athlete Side-Lying 1

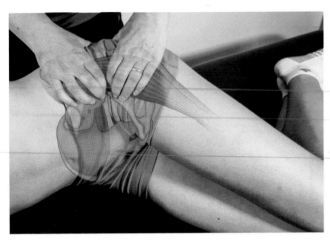

1. *Athlete is side-lying with hips and knees flexed*
2. *Stand behind athlete and slowly sink fingers of both hands into the TFL by curling fingers around the bulk of the tissues.*

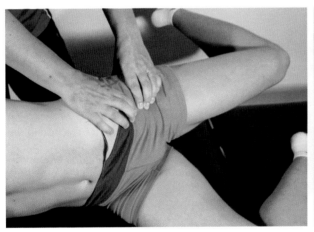 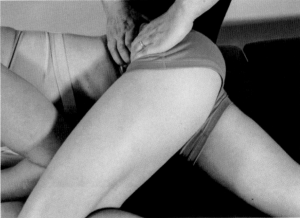

3. *Maintain the depth and position.*
   - *Athlete can then extend the ipsilateral hip slowly to end of range.*
   - *Athlete then flexes hip toward chest.*
4. *Remove hands and repeat step 2, this time moving the fingers distally.*

Soft-Tissue Treatment: Athlete Side-Lying 2

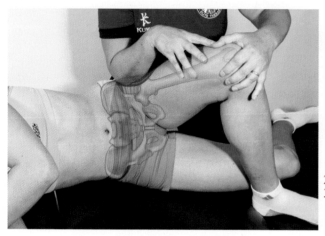

1. Athlete is side-lying with hips and knees flexed.
2. Stand behind athlete.
3. Passively flex and externally rotate the ipsilateral hip and place the foot just anterior to the contralateral knee.

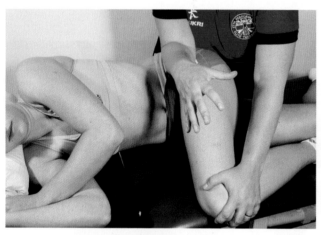

4. Maintain contact with the ipsilateral knee, taking the weight.
5. Sink into the tissues of the TFL using the elbow.
6. Athlete actively adducts hip, lowering the knee to the plinth.

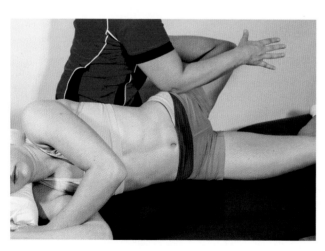

7. Ask the athlete to relax, and passively externally rotate and extend the ipsilateral hip.
8. Repeat this process until all of the tissues have been addressed.

Dry Needling for Tensor Fascia Latae

Dry needling should only be performed by a qualified and insured physical therapist, owing to the invasive nature of the technique and serious anatomical considerations.

1. Note the referral pattern—does this represent your athlete's pain?
2. Athlete is supine or side-lying.
3. Locate TP, palpating for taut band.
4. Needle perpendicularly to the muscle tissues, directly into the trigger point or taut band.

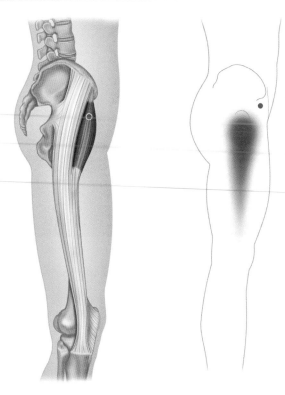

Figure 6.45: TFL trigger points and referral pattern

Muscle Energy Techniques (MET) of TFL and ITT: Athlete Supine

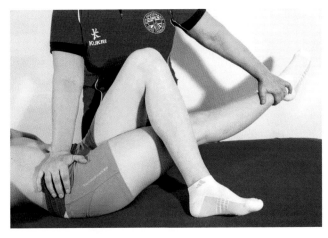

1. *Determine the length of tissues using the modified Ober's test.*
2. *Athlete is supine with contralateral knee flexed and crossed over the ipsilateral leg, with foot resting on the plinth.*
3. *Contact the contralateral knee (lateral aspect), and hold the ipsilateral lower leg just above the ankle*
4. *Then adduct the ipsilateral leg passively, until you feel resistance.*
5. *Athlete abducts hip against your resistance using approximately twenty percent of their overall strength for ten to twelve seconds.*
6. *Utilizing the PIR period (approximately twenty seconds), take the ipsilateral femur further into adduction.*
7. *Repeat these steps until no further gains are achieved.*

Additional Treatment Considerations: MET for Rectus Femoris—Athlete Prone

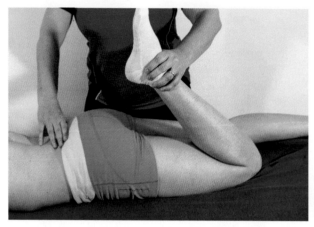

1. Athlete is prone.
2. Athlete's knee is passively flexed until you feel resistance
3. Athlete extends knee against your resistance using approximately twenty percent of overall strength for ten to twelve seconds.

4. Utilizing the PIR period (approximately twenty seconds), take knee into further flexion.
5. Repeat these steps until no further gains are achieved.

SIJ Mobilizations

Grading Information Box

- Grade I—small-amplitude movement at the beginning of the available range
- Grade II—large-amplitude movement within the available range of movement
- Grade III—large-amplitude movement that reaches the end of the range of movement
- Grade VI—small-amplitude movement at the very end of the range of movement
- Grade V—high-velocity thrust.

Assessment for Anterior Rotation of the Ilium

Place fingers on ASIS and PSIS of the ipsilateral side.
- *ASIS slightly lower than the PSIS = normal*
- *ASIS much lower than the PSIS in comparison to the other side = anterior rotation*
  - *Ensure all advised soft-tissue work is done*
  - *Reassess*
- *If pelvis is still anteriorly rotated, mobilize into posterior rotation.*

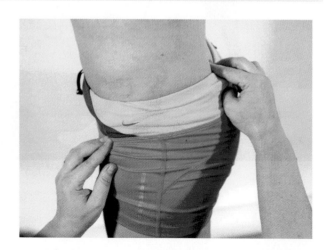

Treatment for Anterior Rotation of the Ilium

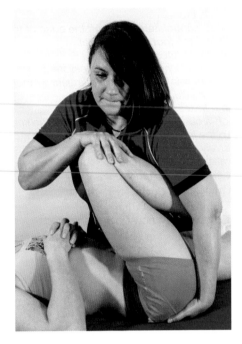
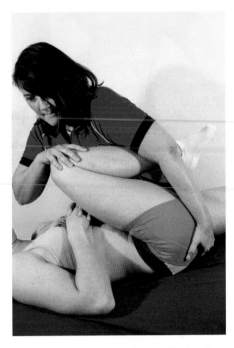

1. *Athlete is supine.*
2. *Stand on the contralateral side, where the athlete's leg is extended.*
3. *Athlete's ipsilateral leg is flexed to ninety degrees and the knee is flexed.*
4. *Lean over the contralateral leg and reach a hand under the ipsilaterally flexed hip, fixing fingers over the posterior structures and ischial tuberosity.*
5. *Place the heel of your hand on the ipsilateral ASIS.*

6. *Take the athlete's hip into further flexion by pulling on the ischial tuberosity and surrounding tissues, simultaneously pushing the ASIS backward and downward.*
   - *Grade I/II for pain, III/IV for stiffness.*
7. *An MET process can now be implemented.*
   - *Athlete extends against your resistance.*
8. *This can also be done with the athlete side-lying.*

Assessment for Posterior Rotation of the Ilium

Place your fingers on ASIS and PSIS of the ipsilateral side.
- *ASIS slightly lower than the PSIS = normal*
- *PSIS lower than the ASIS or both level in comparison to the other side = posterior rotation of the ilium*
  - *Ensure all advised soft-tissue work is done*
  - *Reassess*
- *If pelvis is still posteriorly rotated, mobilize into anterior rotation.*

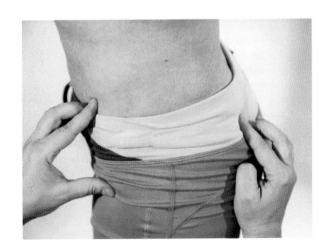

Treatment for Posterior Rotation of the Ilium

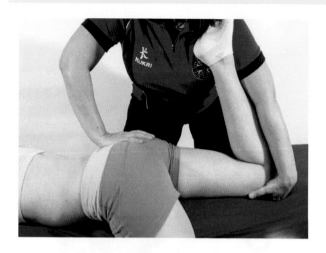

1. *Athlete is prone.*
2. *Athlete's contralateral leg is off the edge of the plinth and the foot is on the floor.*
3. *Stand on ipsilateral side.*
4. *Place heel of one hand on the ipsilateral (same side as anterior rotation) PSIS, with fingers wrapping around the ilium.*
5. *Athlete flexes ipsilateral knee.*
6. *Reach around to the lateral surface of the knee, grasp the leg just above the knee.*
7. *Passively extend the hip whilst pushing forward and upward on the PSIS (find the direction where the joint moves more freely).*
   - Grade I/II for pain, III/IV for stiffness.
   - Mobilize edge of ilium
8. *MET process can now be implemented.*
   - Athlete adds hip flexion against resistance.

Mobilizing the SIJ

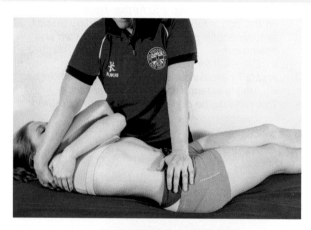

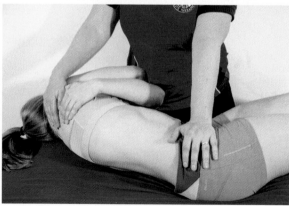

1. *Athlete is supine.*
2. *Athlete's arms are folded across the chest.*
3. *The contralateral leg is crossed over the ipsilateral leg (same side as SIJ to be mobilized).*

4. *The torso side is flexed toward the SIJ to be mobilized.*
5. *Take bilateral legs over toward the side to be mobilized.*
6. *Athlete is now in banana position.*
7. *Rotate athlete's trunk away from the SIJ to be treated (toward the contralateral side) and hold this position.*
8. *Place the heel of your hand onto the ipsilateral ASIS and direct pressure posteriorly.*
   - Grade I/II for pain, III/IV for stiffness.
9. *An MET process can now be implemented.*
   - Athlete attempts to rotate toward the SIJ and simultaneously rotates the pelvis toward the midline.
   - Offer resistance at both points.

SIJ Home Advice

The home mobilization exercises below are very effective at maintaining the athlete's pelvic position until the therapist sees them again. Once the pelvis is able to maintain its position, strengthening exercises should be introduced to re-establish force closure.

1. Stretch both sides (a) and (b).
2. Contract abdominal muscles when in supine position (b).

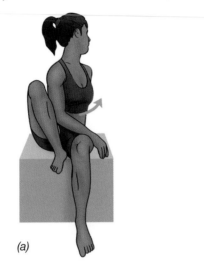

(a)

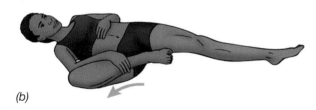

(b)

Figure 6.46: Self correction for SIJ stiffness

1. Athlete pushes femur caudad (toward the foot) with enough force to elevate the buttock off the plinth.
2. Athlete flexes neck and lifts head to activate abdominal structures.
3. Repeat five times on both sides throughout the day.

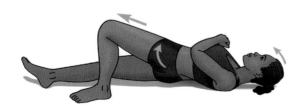

Figure 6.47: Self traction in supine position

1. Athlete pushes one knee forward and pulls the other back toward the back of the seat.
   - Abdominal structures must be activated to pull the pelvis upward (posterior rotation).
2. Repeat five times on both sides throughout the day.

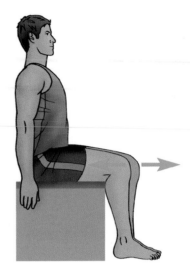

Figure 6.48: Self traction in sitting position

1. Athlete places ipsilateral foot against the doorframe.
2. Abdominal structures are activated to encourage posterior rotation.
3. Athlete pushes foot against the doorframe (isometric contraction).
4. Minimal movement is allowed.
5. Athlete holds the contraction for five to ten seconds.
6. This is repeated for both sides.

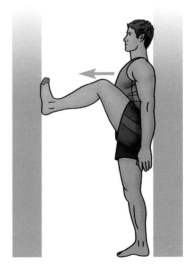

Figure 6.49: Isometric self correction

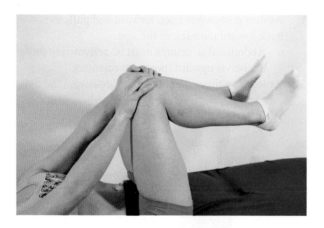

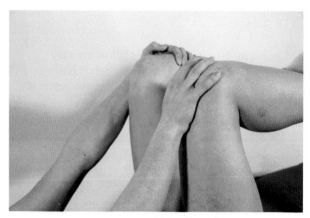

1. *Athlete is in supine position, hips and knees flexed in ninety degrees.*
2. *Athlete places one hand just superior to one knee (right shown).*
   - *Flexes hip against own resistance.*
3. *Athlete places other hand just distal to other knee (left shown).*
   - *Extends hip against own resistance.*

4. *Athlete performs both (2) and (3) above simultaneously, holding for twenty seconds.*

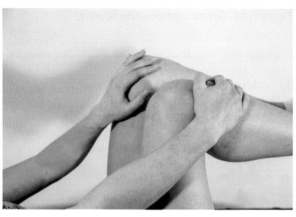

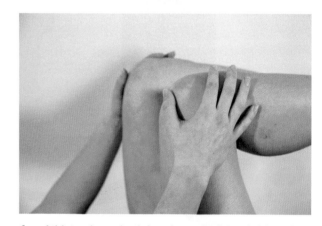

5. *Athlete repeats points (1–4) above after swapping the hands over.*

6. *Athlete places both hands on the lateral sides of knees.*
   - *Abducts against own resistance.*

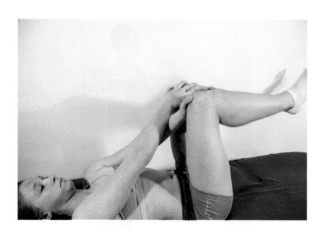

7. *Athlete crosses over hands and places them on the medial sides of both knees.*
   - *Adducts against own resistance.*

Stretching Exercises to Support Treatment Outcomes

With the following important observations. Static stretching:

1. Is good for sports requiring lots of flexibility (gymnastics, dance).
2. For less than sixty seconds does not compromise maximal muscle performance (Kay and Blazevich, 2012).
3. Should not be performed immediately prior to competitions unless strategically placed at the beginning of a warm-up program (Taylor et al., 2009).
4. Longer stretches for ninety seconds and more engage the fascial structures (Muller and Schleip, 2013).
   - Reduce edema
   - Increase hydrostatic balance of tissues (Schleip and Müller, 2013).

---

1. Athlete is on hands and knees.
2. Positions knee over the edge of the plinth, hooking foot over contralateral leg for support.
3. Stretches ipsilateral femur fully below the edge of the plinth.
   - Holds for five seconds
   - Lifts higher than the edge of the plinth for five seconds.
4. This is repeated both sides ten times.

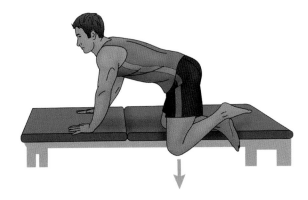

Figure 6.50: SIJ stretch

1. Athlete places foot on a chair or stool.
2. Flexes the lumbar, thoracic, and cervical spine.
3. Rotates away from the hip allowing the ipsilateral arm to lie inside the ipsilateral knee.
4. This stretch is held for thirty to ninety seconds, allowing time for fascial involvement if necessary (as described below).

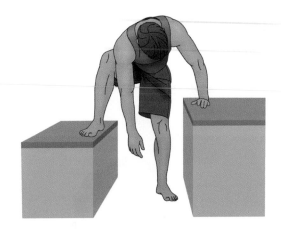

Figure 6.51: Stretch for right anterior rotation of the ilium

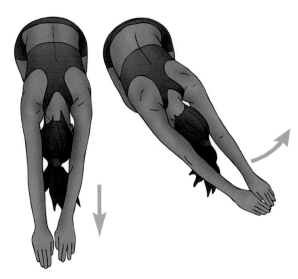

Figure 6.52: Stretches for latissimus dorsi

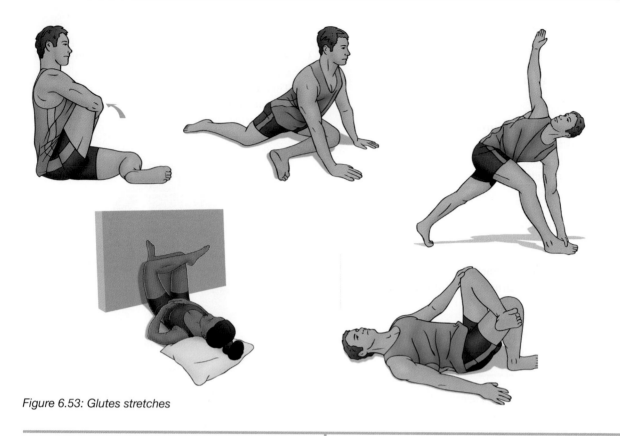

Figure 6.53: Glutes stretches

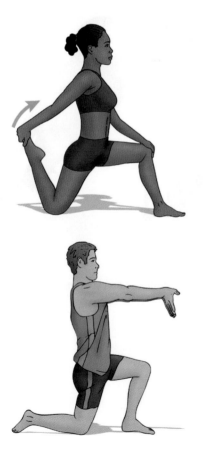

Figure 6.54: Psoas stretches

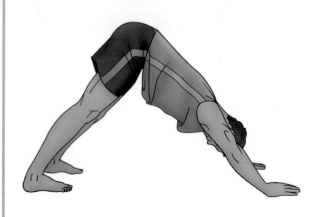

Figure 6.55: Superficial back line (SBL) stretch / Downward dog

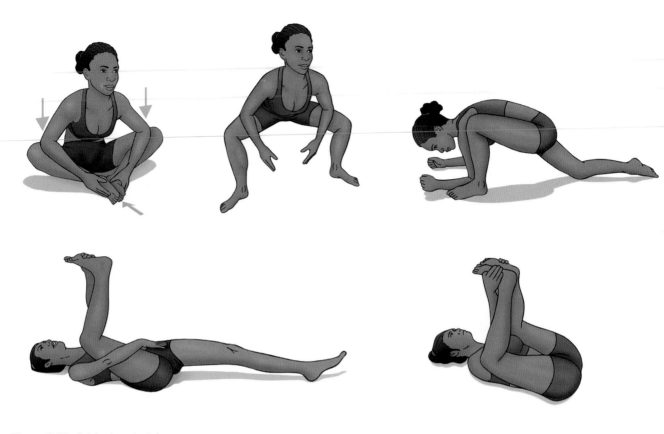

Figure 6.56: Adductor stretches

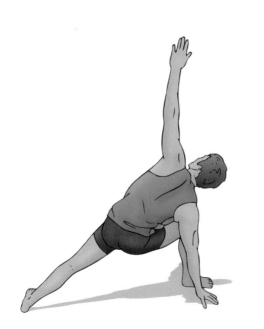

Figure 6.57: TFL and spiral line stretch

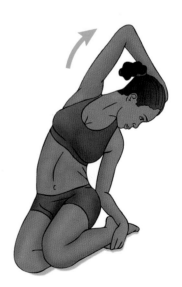

Figure 6.58: QL stretch

Strengthening Exercises Following SIJ Dysfunction

Squatting

Please ensure that you have assessed the squat fully as described in Chapter 5 prior to prescribing the exercises described below. These exercises are too basic for elite athletes.

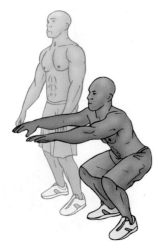

Figure 6.59: Basic bodyweight squat

Squat Progressions

1. Begin with mini-squats (picture 2 below) if the squat assessment produces faulty movement patterns or causes discomfort.
   - Mini-squat
   - Ten to fifteen reps, three sets, three times a day.
2. Progress to mini-squats with holds (picture 3 below).
   - Mini-squat then hold for five to ten seconds
   - Return to neutral
   - Ten to fifteen reps, three sets, three times a day.
3. Progress to deeper squats (picture 4 below).
   - Mini-squat then hold
   - Deeper squat then hold
   - Return to mini-squat then hold
   - Return to neutral
   - Ten to fifteen reps, three sets, three times a day.

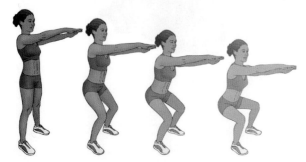

Figure 6.60: Squatting progressions

Single-Leg Squat

Assessment: Please ensure you assess for all the anomalies shown in Figures 6.60–6.61 before prescribing the single-leg squat. This can also be used as an outcome measure. Begin with mini-squats as above until strength and quality have returned.

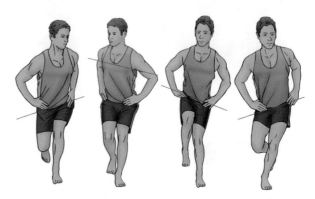

Figure 6.61: Movement compensations when performing a single-leg squat

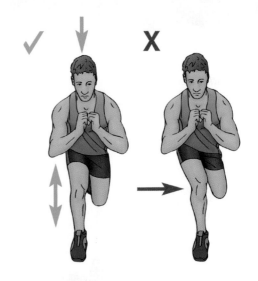

Figure 6.62: Demonstration of movement compensations when performing a single-leg squat

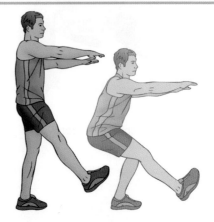

Figure 6.63: Single-leg squat exercise

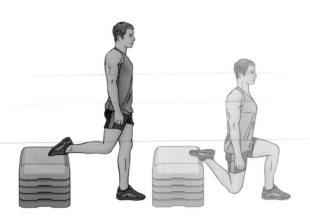

Figure 6.64: Split squat exercise

Plank Position

1. This can be performed on elbows or hands.
2. If this is too difficult, have your athlete start on the anterior surface of the knees, ensuring that the body is still kept in the plank position.
3. Hold for as long as possible.
   - The body should form a straight line from shoulders to ankles
   - No rotation is allowed
   - No sinking into lumbar extension
   - Head remains in neutral.
4. Begin with small sets of three reps of ten seconds, and build from there.
5. When able to hold position for an extended period of time, attempt extending one leg approximately forty degrees and holding, then repeat with the other side.
   - Ensure that the compensatory patterns above do not occur.

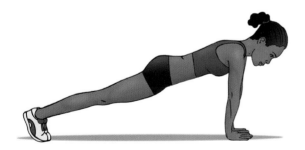

Figure 6.65: Plank position

Side Plank Position

1. Ensure that the body, neck, and head are all in neutral.
2. Ensure that the athlete's elbow is directly under the shoulder.
   - The body should form a straight line from the head to the feet
   - No rotation is allowed
   - No sinking into lumbar side flexion
   - Head remains in neutral.
3. Begin with small sets of three reps of ten seconds, and build from there.
4. When able to hold position for an extended period of time, attempt abducting arm to ninety degrees and abducting leg to approximately forty-five degrees at the same time.
   - Ensure that the compensatory patterns above do not occur.

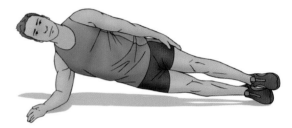

Figure 6.66: Side plank position

Bridge Assessment

Assess the bridge position first to ensure that there are no compensatory patterns:

- Rotation
- Shaking
- Hips dipping one side or the other
- Unable to hold straight-line position

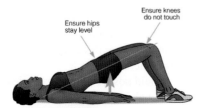

Figure 6.67: Bridge position

Gluteus Medius Exercise

1. Ensure bridge assessment is completed.
2. Raise the upper leg, until just before the hip rotates backward, to a count of five.
3. Hold this position for a count of five.
4. Lower to a count of five.
5. Twenty reps, three sets, three times a day.
6. Progressions:
   - Progress to forty reps.
   - Add Thera-Band around the knees.
   - Athlete can hold weight on the outer leg.
   - Outer leg can be extended and internally rotated.

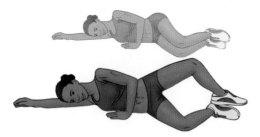

Figure 6.68: Gluteus medius exercise

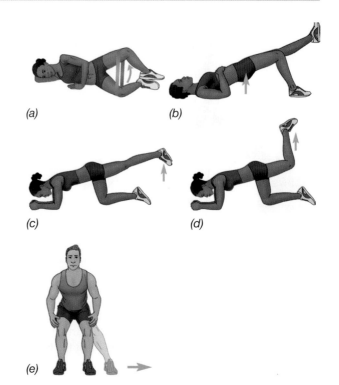

Figure 6.70: Hip exercises. (a) Clam exercise: using a band for additional resistance. (b) Single-leg bridge: athlete adopts the position shown, ensure no compensatory patterns as mentioned above. (c and d) Hip extension exercises on all fours: while on hands and knees, extend one leg upward. This exercise can be done with the leg straight (harder) or with the knee bent (easier). (e) Side-step exercise: while in a slight squat position, take small steps sideways while keeping your toes pointed forward

References

Gibbons SCT, Pelley B, and Molgaard J (2001) Biomechanics and stability mechanisms of psoas major. Proceedings of 4th Interdisciplinary World Conference on Low Back Pain, Montreal, Canada, November 9–11, 2001

Kay A and Blazevich A (2012) Effect of acute static stretch on maximal muscle performance. Medicine and *Science in Sports and Exercise* 44(1): 154–164

Muller DG and Schleip R (2013) Fascial fitness: fascia oriented training for bodywork and movement therapies. Terra Rosa e-magazine 7. Available online at: http://www.somatics.de/FascialFitnessTerraRosa.pdf. (Accessed June 2015)

Palastanga N and Soames R (2012) *Anatomy and Human Movement: Structure and Function.* Edinburgh: Churchill Livingstone

Schleip R and Müller DG (2013) Training principles for fascial connective tissues: scientific foundation and suggested practical applications. *Journal of Bodywork and Movement Therapies* 17(1): 103–115

Takazakura R, Takahashi M, Nitta N, and Murata K (2004) Diaphragmatic motion in the sitting and supine positions: healthy subject study using a vertically open magnetic resonance system. *Journal of Magnetic Resonance Imaging* 19: 605–609

Taylor K, Sheppard J, Lee H, and Plummer N (2009) Negative effect of static stretching restored when combined with a sport specific warm-up component. *Journal of Science and Medicine in Sport* 12(6): 657–661

An athlete presenting with piriformis syndrome (PS) will describe pain in the buttock (sciatic-notch area— Figure 7.1) or in the lower back, with or without sciatic-nerve irritation (sciatic-nerve entrapment/radicular pain), and clinically there will be a hypertrophied piriformis muscle (Shapiro and Preston, 2009). These signs and symptoms become more apparent particularly when the athlete sits for prolonged periods of time on a hard surface (Shapiro and Preston, 2009). In fact, intolerance to sitting like this is probably the clearest indicator (Papadopoulos and Khan, 2004).

Primary PS is a neuromuscular condition causing buttock pain, which may or may not include some radicular pain, generally caused by anatomical anomalies of the muscle itself. Secondary PS (more common than primary) is related to trauma, with associated ischemia, traction of the muscle or nerve, changes in muscle strength or flexibility, and biomechanical misalignment of the lower extremity, all of which make lower-extremity assessment extremely important.

Typically, people with this condition present with:

- A pronated foot (see Figure 7.2b) on the ipsilateral side
- A functional leg-length discrepancy (see Figure 7.3), where usually the affected side is the long side
- Tight external hip rotators and adductors on the ipsilateral side
- Weak hip abductors on the ipsilateral side.

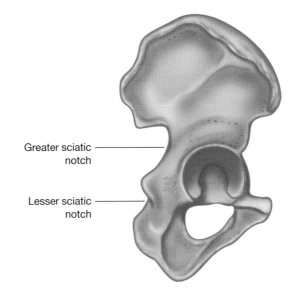

Greater sciatic notch

Lesser sciatic notch

Figure 7.1: The sciatic notch

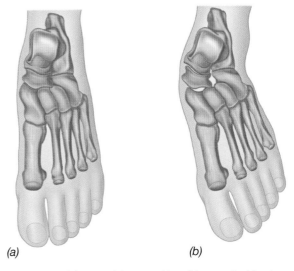

(a)   (b)

Figure 7.2: (a) normal foot position (b) pronated foot

Adducting and medially rotating the hip joint (increasing piriformis muscle tension), unsurprisingly, has been shown to increase the athlete's pain (Papadopoulos and Khan, 2004; Shapiro and Preston, 2009; Hopayian et al., 2010). Commonly there is also an increased Q angle (Figure 7.4), and/or a valgus knee position (Figure 7.5).

Common anomalies observed when assessing gait:

- Overpronation in late midstance ensures the femur medially rotates when lateral rotation is demanded.
- The pelvis rotates externally in the swing phase on the contralateral leg, encouraging shearing stresses to travel cephalad into the femur.
- Increased tension in the piriformis muscle causes subsequent compression of the sciatic nerve.

Compression of the sciatic nerve may cause varied neurological symptoms in the lower extremity. However, with piriformis syndrome, neurological testing typically doesn't show any true neuropathy or radicular injury. Deep tendon reflexes, sensation, and muscle strength are not usually affected.

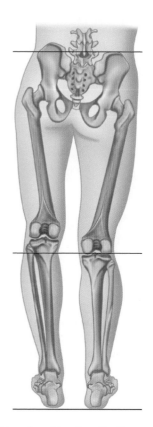

Figure 7.3: Functional leg-length discrepancy. The affected side in this example would typically be the left-hand side

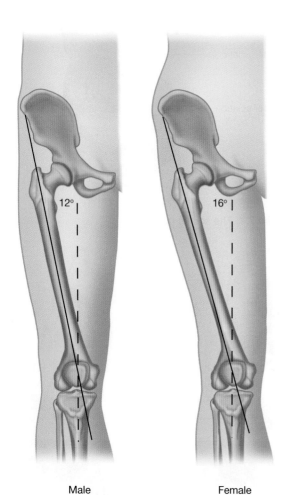

Male   Female

Figure 7.4: Comparison of the male and female Q angle

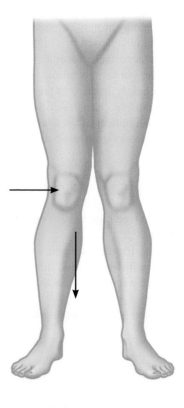

Figure 7.5: Valgus knee position

Piriformis

Attachments

- Piriformis arises from the periosteal fascia surrounding the anterior S2–S4
- It travels between and lateral to the anterior sacral foramina
- There is an additional attachment from the periosteal fascia surrounding the gluteal surface of the ilium and the pelvic surface of the sacrotuberous ligament
- It passes out of the pelvis through the greater sciatic foramen into the gluteal region
- Fibers continue to pass downward, laterally, and forward, narrowing into a tendon, which invests into the upper border and medial side of the periosteal fascia surrounding the greater trochanter of the femur.

Innervation

- Anterior rami of the sacral plexus (root value L5, S1, and S2)
- Skin covering this area (L5, S1, and S2).

Action

- Anatomical position—lateral rotator of the femur
- Holds head of femur in the acetabulum
- In sitting becomes an abductor
  - Sliding along a bench without standing up
  - Taking the legs out of the car prior to standing up
- Stabilizes the pelvis when the trunk is rotated
- Controls the balance of the pelvis when standing on a moving bus.

Antagonists

- Hip extended: gluteus medius, gluteus minimus (medial rotators).

Synergists

- When hip is flexed and abducted:
  - Middle fibers of gluteus maximus (GM)
  - Gluteus medius, gluteus minimus
  - Tensor fascia latae (TFL)
  - Sartorius
- Abduction is opposed by all of the adductors (antagonists), lower fibers of GM, psoas major, and the iliacus.

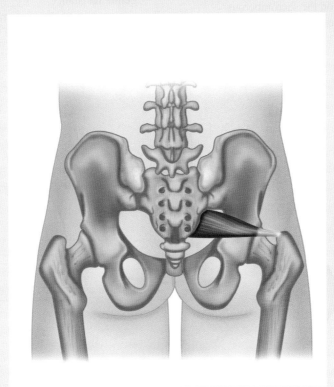

Figure 7.6: Piriformis

There are many signs and symptoms of piriformis syndrome, most commonly an increase in pain somewhere around the muscles' fascial attachments after sitting for longer than fifteen to twenty minutes, as already mentioned (Boyajian et al., 2008):

- Pain +/– paresthesia radiating from sacrum to gluteal area, posterior thigh, just above the knee (Foster, 2002; DiGiovanna et al., 2005)
- Walking reduces the pain
- No movement increases the pain
- Contralateral SIJ pain
- Pain when rising from sitting or squatting positions
- Changing positions does not resolve pain completely
- Difficulty walking (antalgic gait or foot drop)
- Weakness in lower limb (ipsilateral)
- Numbness in foot (ipsilateral).

A hypertonic piriformis muscle creates ipsilateral external rotation of the hip (look out for this sign when the athlete is lying relaxed in supine position). Active attempts at placing the foot in a midline position often result in pain (Frieberg and Vinke, 2008).

Sacral torsion (often ipsilateral anterior rotation on a contralateral oblique axis) following spasm of the piriformis contributes to compensatory rotation of the lower lumbar vertebrae in the opposing direction (double crush) (see Figure 7.7). The compensatory unaccustomed stress placed on the sacrotuberous ligament may lead to compression of the pudendal nerves, or an increase in mechanical stress on the innominates resulting in groin or pelvic pain (Chaitow, 1988). Referral to Chapter 5 on assessment of SIJ dysfunction will help rule out "double-crush" syndrome.

MRI (magnetic resonance imaging), CT (computed tomography), EMG (electromyography), and ultrasound are useful in excluding conditions that produce similar symptoms to piriformis syndrome. The presence of sciatic nerve irritation can be detected by magnetic resonance neurography, but that is rarely required.

Palpation

The piriformis muscle is located deep to the gluteus maximus (GM) and in most cases superficial to the sciatic nerve.

1. Athlete is in prone position.
2. Locate the coccyx, posterior superior iliac spine (PSIS), and the greater trochanter.
3. Draw an imaginary line from the PSIS to the coccyx, then another from the greater trochanter, perpendicular to the line above.
4. The piriformis lies along the perpendicular line.
5. Palpate through the GM (remembering what was discussed in Chapter 2: Fascia).
6. To confirm location, athlete flexes knee to ninety degrees and laterally rotates hip as you provide gentle resistance.
7. Contraction of the piriformis muscle can be felt deep to the contraction of the GM.

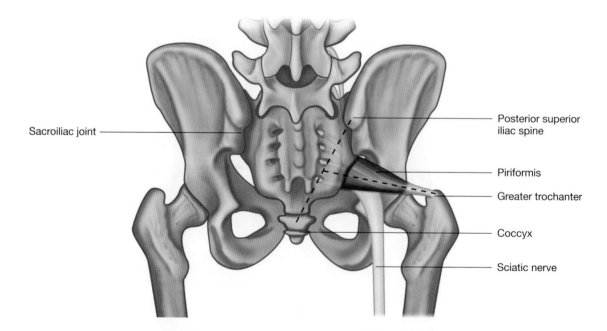

Figure 7.7: The "double-crush" pain at the SIJ and piriformis

Sacroiliac joint

Posterior superior iliac spine

Piriformis

Greater trochanter

Coccyx

Sciatic nerve

Testing

You will have performed a comprehensive subjective assessment and, in the objective stage, will have included lumbar spine and pelvic assessments, muscle length and strength relationships, joint ranges of movement, and muscle firing sequences (these can be found in Chapter 5: SIJ Dysfunction—Assessment). When your assessments and clinical reasoning identify piriformis syndrome, manual-therapy techniques to reduce/relieve neural compression can begin.

The FAIR Test

Of the many diagnostic techniques, the "flexion adduction internal rotation" (FAIR) technique shows the highest specificity[1] (0.881) and sensitivity[2] (0.832), particularly when used in combination with functional electromyography examination (Fishman et al., 2002; Filler et al., 2005; Hopayian et al., 2010; Kean Chen and Nizar, 2012). Tenderness at the gluteal region around the piriformis muscle (Lasègue sign) has been noted to be the most consistent clinical finding in piriformis syndrome (Durrani and Winnie, 1991).

1. Athlete is in supine position.
2. Stand on contralateral side of athlete.
3. Passively flex athlete's hip to sixty degrees and knee to ninety degrees.
4. Stabilize ipsilateral hip.
5. Internally rotate and adduct athlete's hip by applying downward pressure onto the knee (see Figure 7.8).
6. The FAIR test result is positive if buttock pain is reproduced.

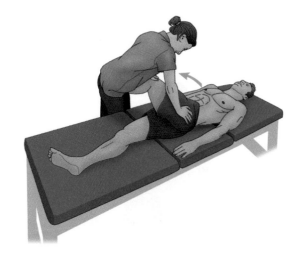

Figure 7.8: The FAIR test for piriformis syndrome

---

1. The ability of a test to correctly classify an individual as disease-free is called the test's specificity. The best possible specificity score is 1.0, where 100% of people without the condition are correctly identified as such by the test. Also called the true negative rate.
2. Sensitivity is the ability of a test to correctly classify an individual as "diseased." Again, the best possible score would be 1.0, where 100% of people who have the disease are correctly identified as such by the test. Also called the true positive rate.

Piriformis Length Test 1

1. Athlete is in supine relaxed position.
2. Observe the position of the feet: is one more externally rotated than the other?

Piriformis Length Test 2

1. Athlete is prone.
2. Flex athlete's knee to ninety degrees and hold the ipsilateral foot.
3. Stabilize the ipsilateral pelvis.
4. Passively internally rotate athlete's ipsilateral hip and compare to the contralateral side.
5. Any reduction in range indicates a shortening of the piriformis.

Piriformis Length Test 3

1. Athlete is prone.
2. Athlete flexes both knees to ninety degrees, keeping the knees together.
3. Athlete then allows the hips to internally rotate by allowing the feet to fall outward slowly.
4. Note any difference in range between left and right.
5. The side that stays more perpendicular to the plinth is indicative of a short piriformis muscle.

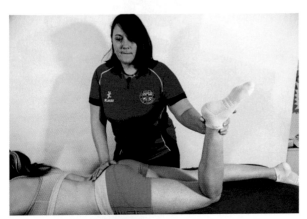

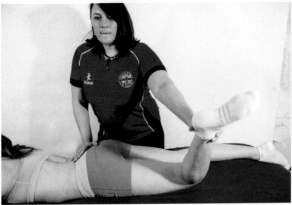

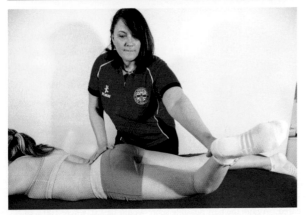

Treatment

Just to reiterate, prior to any therapy input, and because there can be similar symptoms in differing pathology, it is imperative that a complete and thorough evaluation is performed (and that there is awareness of differential diagnoses) in an attempt to reproduce the athlete's symptoms. Reading Chapter 2 on fascia and its global influence on the body both in health and in illness will help you to appreciate that when one part of the body is injured (cut surgically, torn, fractured, infected, inflamed, etc.), compensatory patterns occur.

NB: No injury occurs in isolation; with all injuries, the body finds ways of adapting in order that it can continue to function.

Compensatory or facilitative mechanisms in people with piriformis syndrome may show the following:

- Reduced range of movement in the upper thoracic spine
- Tissue texture changes in the thoracic spine around T4
- Lumbosacral pain
- Decreased range of movement of the contralateral C2 and ipsilateral occiput–atlas
- Gastrointestinal disorders
- Headaches.

Conservative treatment may consist of:

- Pain medication
- NSAIDs[3] (Papadopoulos and Khan, 2004; Shapiro and Preston, 2009)
- Correction of biomechanical abnormalities (Brukner and Khan, 2014)
- Specific stretching (Papadopoulos and Khan, 2004; Shapiro and Preston, 2009)
- Soft-tissue therapy (Brukner and Khan, 2014)
  - Massage to help decrease pain and spasm, and reduce related strain in other parts of the body
  - Instrument-assisted techniques
  - Dynamic taping
- Lifestyle modifications to reduce joint/muscle irritation (Byrd, 2005)
- Acupuncture; dry needling to help reduce spasm and help toward restoring passive range of movement (ROM) (Brukner and Khan, 2014)
- Botulinum toxin injections followed by stretching (Fishman et al., 2002)
- Physical therapy (Papadopoulos and Khan, 2004; Shapiro and Preston, 2009)

- Neurodynamic techniques
- Pelvic and spinal realignment
- Joint mobilization to restore full range of passive movement
- Strengthening programs for the whole body (Pilates)
- Proprioception exercises
- Biomechanical analysis
- Agility and sports-specific assessments and exercises (address over-striding while running)
- Adjunct core-stability exercise program (Byrd, 2005; Cramp et al., 2007).
- Shoe assessment.

However, there do not appear to be any comprehensive guidelines available regarding the most effective conservative management of this condition. It is also worth mentioning that, should conservative treatment fail, injection or surgical releases are more advanced options (Papadopoulos and Khan, 2004; Shapiro and Preston, 2009).

Manual Therapy

So, where do we start? Before moving forward with the suggestions below, take a moment to really think about what is happening in the body when a structure is so dysfunctional that it is causing pain and altered ROM or gait (as discussed previously), and remind yourself how the body adapts to this dysfunction by spreading the load and causing further dysfunction/pain.

Ask yourself the questions: How did the piriformis become like this? Is it a primary condition or a secondary adaptation due to factors such as biomechanical abnormalities, recent training increases with altered gait, a recent ankle sprain, pelvic or lower back pain, shoulder or thoracic dysfunction, etc.?

Soft-tissue techniques vary from therapist to therapist. The ones that I am about to share with you are the ones I find are most effective. I am not attempting to belittle or put aside other techniques, or encouraging you to change your current practice; I am simply introducing these techniques as additional tools for your ever-growing toolbox—ideas that you may want to consider if you are not getting the results you require.

I would recommend addressing any SIJ or sacral obliquity first (see Chapter 5), followed by targeted soft-tissue work to each muscle that has a direct or indirect relationship with the piriformis muscle.

---

3. Nonsteroidal anti-inflammatory drugs.

Gluteus Maximus (GM)

Full detailed anatomy can be found in Chapter 6 (see page 83).

GM originates from the fascia surrounding the gluteal surface of the ilium and sacrum, the lumbar fascia, and the sacrotuberous ligament. It invests into the periosteum of the gluteal tuberosity of the femur and the iliotibial tract, and is innervated by the inferior gluteal nerve (L5, S1, and S2 nerve roots).

Use the following techniques to encourage relaxation of the fascial attachments (see also Chapter 6). Never work outside your patient's level of discomfort (remember your VAS[4])!

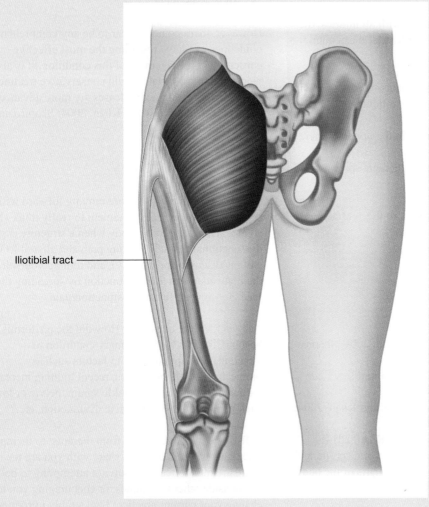

Iliotibial tract ——

Figure 7.9: Gluteus maximus

---

4. VAS—visual analogue scale (see Glossary, Chapter 1).

Soft-Tissue Treatment: Athlete Prone

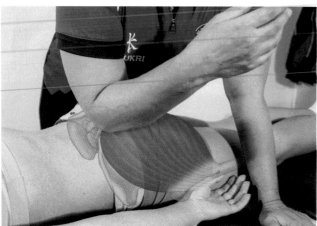

1. *This technique can be done through clothing.*
2. *Athlete's feet are over the edge of the plinth.*
3. *Loosen up the muscle bulk using kneading/ compression-type techniques.*
4. *Place an elbow just below the PSIS and lateral to the sacral ridge, and sink slowly into the tissues at a speed that they allow (fascial sink), at a level no more than 6/10 VAS (Hawker et al., 2011).*
5. *Maintain pressure until the discomfort drops to approximately 2/10.*
6. *Athlete drops the ipsilateral pelvis (downward tilt).*
7. *Lift the elbow and move to a position approximately half an inch distal to the starting point and repeat.*
8. *Continue until you are adjacent to S5.*
9. *Now, using the same technique, work just under the iliac crest and travel laterally for approximately four inches.*

Soft-Tissue Treatment: Athlete Side-Lying 1

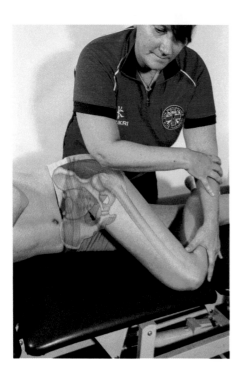

1. *This technique can be done through clothing.*
2. *Locate the greater trochanter.*
3. *Place an elbow above the most superior portion and adopt the "fascial sink".*
4. *Athlete gently tilts the pelvis backward and forward, then laterally up and down.*
5. *Move around the spherical surface of the greater trochanter in an anticlockwise direction, repeating the pelvic movements.*

Soft-Tissue Treatment: Athlete Side-Lying 2

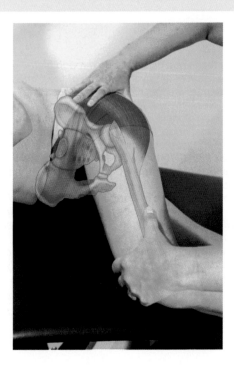

1. *Upper knee and hip are flexed approximately forty-five degrees.*
2. *Face cephalad with foot of athlete's upper leg against your outer thigh.*
   - *Visualize the muscle bulk and, using either the heel of your hand/forearm or thumbs with hand as overpressure, sink into the tissues (lock).*
   - *Ensure no more than 6/10 VAS.*
   - *Wait for the VAS to drop to 2/10.*

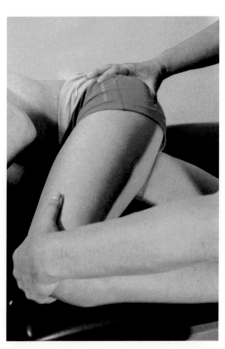

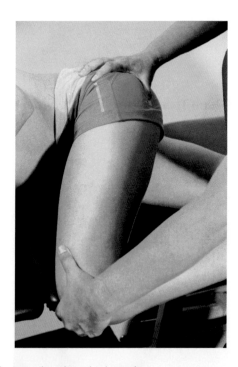

3. *Passively flex the athlete's hip and knee by lunging forward.*
   - *Facilitate the movement by travelling with the tissues*
   - *Stretch the tissues by locking away from the movement (pin and stretch)*
   - *Repeat until the muscle bulk is covered.*
4. *Locate the gluteal tuberosity.*
   - *Engage the tissues surrounding the gluteal tuberosity.*
5. *Lunge forward, taking the hip into deeper flexion.*
   - *Add slow and gentle adduction.*
6. *Reassess using the FAIR test.*

Quadratus Femoris

Attachments

- Situated below the gemellus inferior and above the upper margin of adductor magnus
- Flat quadrilateral muscle, separated from the hip joint by the obturator externus
- Lower fibers emerge from the periosteum and fascia surrounding the ischial tuberosity, just below the lower rim of the acetabulum
- The fibers pass laterally to invest into the tissues surrounding the quadrate tubercle, situated halfway down the intertrochanteric crest, and the area of bone surrounding it.

Innervation

- Nerve to quadratus femoris, root value L4, L5, and S1.

Action

- In the anatomical position, acts as a lateral rotator of the hip joint
- With the hip flexed, acts as an abductor of the hip.

Functional Activity

- All of the lateral rotators function together in the anatomical position controlling the pelvis, particularly when one foot is off the ground
- Even more so when walking
- The lateral rotators work with the GM and the posterior part of gluteus minimus in producing lateral rotation of the lower limb in the forward swing-through phase of gait
- In sitting, crawling, and turning over when lying down they will, however, have a completely different role, producing abduction of the hip and thereby controlling the movements of the pelvis on the flexed thigh.

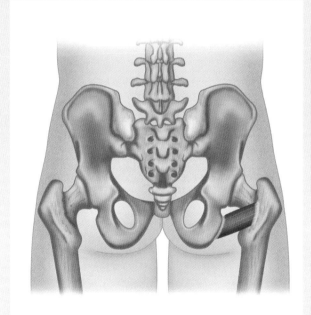

Figure 7.10: Quadratus femoris

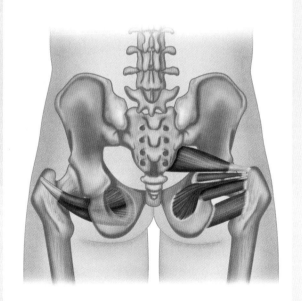

Figure 7.11: Lateral rotators

Soft-Tissue Treatment: Athlete Prone

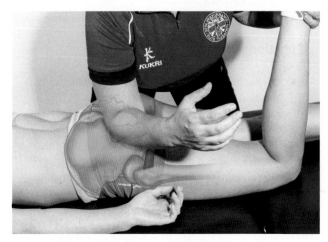

1. *Passively flex the athlete's ipsilateral knee and hold the foot.*
2. *Slowly sink into the tissues between the ischial tuberosity and the greater trochanter (VAS no more than 6/10).*
3. *Wait for VAS 2/10.*

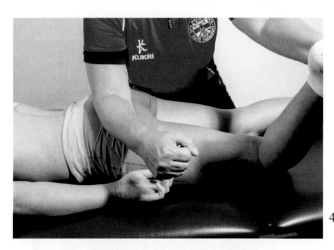

4. *Passively internally rotate the femur using the patient's foot until the VAS increases to 6/10.*

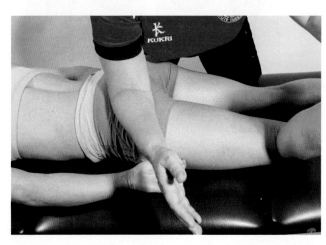

5. *Hold this position until the VAS drops to 2/10.*
6. *Repeat until no further range can be obtained or you are at full ROM.*

Soft-Tissue Treatment: Athlete Standing

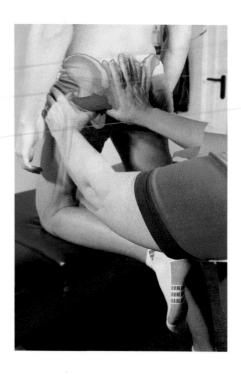

1. *Athlete is standing with ipsilateral knee on plinth or chair.*
2. *Locate the greater trochanter of the femur and slide posterolaterally.*
3. *Maintain pressure or facilitate movement.*
4. *Athlete extends hip (keeping the knee on the chosen surface).*

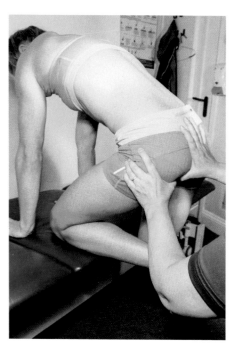

5. *Athlete flexes forward, taking hip into external rotation (after approximately sixty degrees of flexion, piriformis becomes an internal rotator).*
6. *Reassess using the FAIR test.*

Dry Needling for Piriformis

1. Athlete is prone or side-lying.
2. Identify the body landmarks (see Palpation section page 168).
3. Identify the location of the trigger points.
4. Depending on the musculature around, use a two- to three-inch (50–75 mm) needle.
5. Needle perpendicularly to the muscle surface at the greater trochanter or just lateral to the sacrum.
6. Direct the needle into the taut band identified by palpation.
7. Avoid the sciatic nerve.

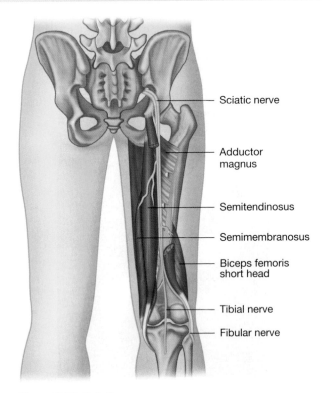

— Sciatic nerve

— Adductor magnus

— Semitendinosus

— Semimembranosus

— Biceps femoris short head

— Tibial nerve

— Fibular nerve

Figure 7.12: Sciatic nerve

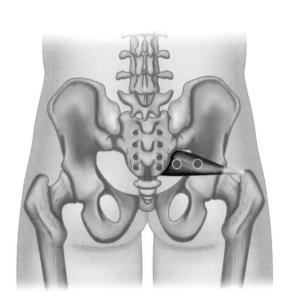

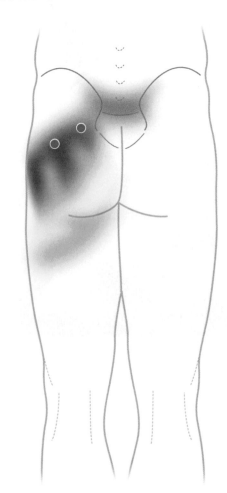

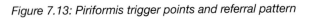

Figure 7.13: Piriformis trigger points and referral pattern

Muscle Energy Techniques (MET): Athlete Supine

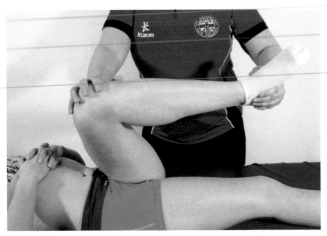

1. Athlete actively flexes the knee on the side that has been assessed as short; hold athlete's foot.
2. Take the leg into internal rotation (where no compensations can be seen in the rest of the body).
3. Hold this position.

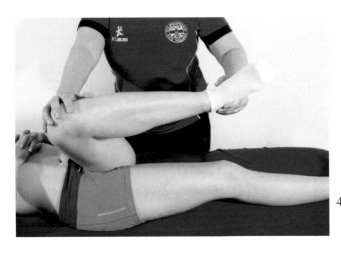

4. Athlete externally rotates femur using approximately twenty to thirty percent of overall strength for ten to twelve seconds.

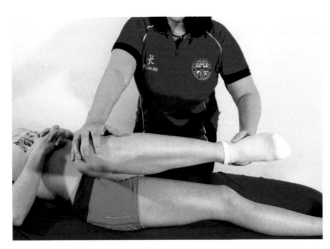

5. Utilizing the post isometric relaxation period (approximately twenty seconds), take the femur further into internal rotation.
6. Repeat this process until:
   - No further gains are achieved
   - Full ROM
   - Prohibited by pain
   - Full body compensation "cheating" begins.

Muscle Energy Techniques (MET): Athlete Prone

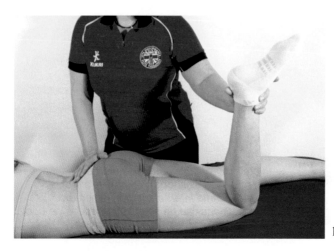

1. Athlete in prone with knee flexed to ninety degrees.

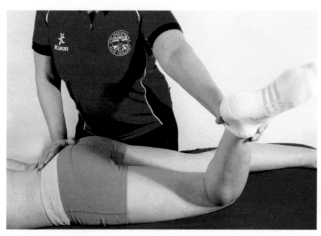

2. Athlete's leg is passively taken into internal rotation until resistance is felt.
3. Athlete externally rotates femur using approximately twenty to thirty percent of overall strength for ten to twelve seconds.

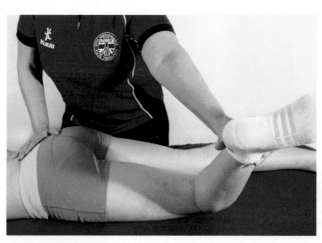

4. Utilizing the post isometric relaxation period (approximately twenty seconds), take the femur further into external rotation.
5. Repeat this process until:
   - No further gains are achieved
   - Full ROM
   - Prohibited by pain
   - Full body compensation "cheating" begins.

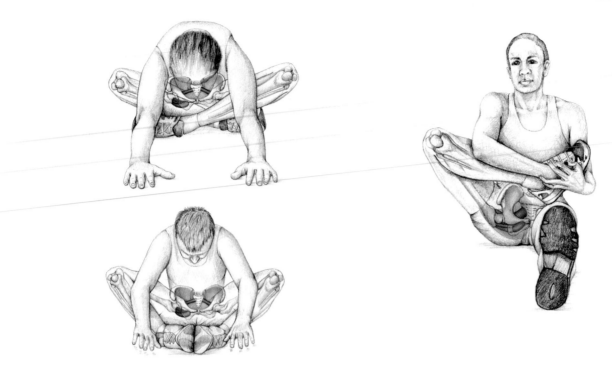

Figure 7.14: Piriformis stretches

References

Boyajian-O'Neill LA, McClain RL, Coleman K, and Thomas PP (2008) Diagnosis and management of piriformis syndrome: an osteopathic approach. *Journal of the American Osteopathic Association* 108(11): 657–664

Brukner P and Khan K (2014) *Clinical Sports Medicine, 4th edition*. London: McGraw-Hill

Byrd JWT (2005) Piriformis syndrome. *Operative Techniques in Sports Medicine* 13: 71–79

Chaitow L (1988) *Soft Tissue Manipulation: A Practitioner's Guide to the Diagnosis and Treatment of Soft-Tissue Dysfunction and Reflex Activity, 3rd edition*. Rochester: Healing Arts Press

Cramp F, Bottrell O, and Campbell H (2007) Non-surgical management of piriformis syndrome: a systematic review. *Physical Therapy Reviews* 12(1): 66–72

DiGiovanna EL, Schiowitz S, and Dowling DJ (2005) *An Osteopathic Approach to Diagnosis and Treatment, 3rd edition*. Philadelphia: Lippincott Williams and Wilkins

Durrani Z and Winnie AP (1991) Piriformis muscle syndrome: an underdiagnosed cause of sciatica. *Journal of Pain and Symptom Management* 6: 374–379

Filler AG, Haynes J, and Jordan SE (2005) Sciatica of non-disc origin and piriformis syndrome: diagnosis by magnetic resonance neurography and interventional magnetic resonance imaging with outcome study of resulting treatment. *Journal of Neurosurgery. Spine* 2: 99–115

Fishman LM, Dombi GW, Michaelsen C, Ringel S, Rozbruch J, and Rosner B (2002) Piriformis syndrome: diagnosis, treatment, and outcome—a 10-year study. *Archives of Physical Medicine and Rehabilitation* 83: 295–301

Foster MR (2002) Piriformis syndrome. *Orthopedics* 25: 821–825

Freiberg AH and Vinke TH (2008) Sciatica and the sacroiliac joint. *Journal of Bone and Joint Surgery. American Volume* 16: 126–136

Hawker GA, Mian S, Kendzerska T, and French M (2011) Measures of pathology and symptoms. *Arthritis Care and Research* 63(11): 240–252

Hopayian K, Song F, Riera R, and Sambandan S (2010) The clinical features of the piriformis syndrome: a systematic review. *European Spine Journal* 19(12): 2095

Kean Chen C and Nizar A (2012) Prevalence of piriformis syndrome in chronic low back pain patients: a clinical diagnosis with modified FAIR test. *Pain Practice* 13(4): 276–281

Palastanga NP and Soames R (2012) *Anatomy and Human Movement: Structure and Function*. Edinburgh: Churchill Livingstone

Papadopoulous EC and Khan SN (2004) Piriformis syndrome and low back pain: a new classification and review of the literature. *Orthopedic Clinics of North America* 35: 65–71

Shapiro BE and Preston DC (2009) Entrapment and compressive neuropathies. *Medical Clinics of North America* 93: 285–315

Appendix: Instrument-Assisted Soft-Tissue Mobilization (IASTM)

Text written and supplied with thanks by Donna Strachan, Kinnective™

What is IASTM?

IASTM is an abbreviation for instrument-assisted soft-tissue manipulation or mobilization. For the purposes of this text mobilization will be attributed, as it can be argued that IASTM achieves more than mobilization alone. This will be discussed later. The term IASTM was coined by Terry Loghmani, who defined it as "The use of a rigid device during soft-tissue manipulation to facilitate the delivery of the mechanical force" (Loghmani and Warden, 2009).

The History of IASTM

IASTM is not a new concept. Indeed, it has been used in many cultures for over 3000 years—e.g. the Chinese *Gua Sha*, which utilizes instruments made from a number of different materials. This includes, though is not limited to, bone, wood, ivory, and jade (Nielsen, 1995). *Strigli* was a technique used by the Romans and Greeks in the second century BC, and utilized ebony, bone, or wooden instruments; *Lomi Lomi* is used in the Hawaiian islands and utilizes wooden logs and sticks (Stillerman, 2009).

IASTM has seen an increase of use in manual therapy in recent years, with the development of stainless steel instruments. The use of stainless steel has revolutionized this technique. The stainless steel provides significantly greater feedback and feel than other materials. When crafted well and used appropriately, IASTM creates a window of insight into the tissues, delivering feel and information about tissues and creating effects that the hands alone simply cannot achieve. This in turn allows for greater clinical insight and ultimately better results achieved with specific and focused treatment.

Kinnective IASTM

The IASTM approach developed by Kinnective is a results-based technique. The premise of this is that the instrument, in conjunction with good technique and appropriate clinical rationale, produces instant results. It has been used in many elite sports in the UK, including by England Rugby, the England Football Association, British Athletics, and at the English Institute of Sport. It was also the chosen instrument supplied to the athletes' village at the London 2012 Olympics. This is because of both the success of the instrument and the use of techniques that have been developed by clinicians who are leading experts in this field. All practitioners have hands, but delivering appropriate manual therapy is full of subtlety and precision that takes years of experience and reflection to develop.

Does It Work?

When used appropriately and with good technique, IASTM is extremely effective at achieving certain results. Clinically these results would be increasing range and improving appropriate muscle function. At a subclinical level it is proposed that cellular function may also be impacted, to improve tissue viability. Ultimately a clinical rationale, however well thought out, is only ever proven or disproven with the results achieved clinically with the individual in question. You make your own evidence. There are a number of ways to do this but Kinnective advocates the "3-rep rule."

The "3-Rep Rule"

Firstly, identify a problematic section of tissue and a direction or movement of involvement. Then choose an outcome measure that challenges the presenting complaint.

For example: the patient presents with a flexion catch in lumbar range of movement (ROM). Examination reveals an area of tension in the thoracolumbar fascia (TLF), which is restricted medially to laterally (M–L). The outcome measure is lumbar flexion. The treatment is IASTM M–L, whilst the individual undergoes lumbar flexion and return to neutral reps in a slow and controlled manner. Whilst engaging the tissues, three repetitions of lumber flexion/neutral are performed and then the patient is asked to "retest" this movement.

Bruising starts with redness, then petechial reaction, and then if you continue you will cause bruising. To avoid bruising, note how quickly these changes occur and adapt your technique to avoid unnecessary bruising.

"Graston" is often used synonymously with IASTM, but remember that you have to be a trained Graston practitioner to use their instruments. If not, you are using IASTM.

If an impact has not been made within two repetitions of the 3-rep rule, this is a sign that treatment is to the wrong area or the wrong rationale is being applied. There will be improvement if the correct structures are being addressed and if this is the appropriate treatment. Without improvement do not continue to treat like this. This approach allows for specific and effective treatment that avoids overworking tissues.

Terminology

It is worth considering the following: "You do what you say you are doing." Consider what you are describing and what is your intent. If you say you are "scraping" the skin, that is what you will do. Would this ever be your intent? This will lead to bruising and skin irritation. Instead, scan the tissues whilst being attentive to the feedback from the instrument so that you may subsequently "engage" the tissues in a constructive manner. Considering the tissues in this manner will impact upon your use of the instrument. Likewise, many people refer to the instruments as "tools." A tool is a blunt implement used for blunt force. An instrument is used for precision and refinement.

What about Bruising?

It should not surprise anyone that if you want to cause bruising, it's much easier if you use a rigid implement. However, this should NOT be synonymous with IASTM. Unless bruising is your goal or an expected and considered outcome, it should not happen. Extensive bruising has been caused by good practitioners who were taught with instruments to "get into" tissues, with significant bruising being the result. Figure A.1 demonstrates deep-seated bruising rather than the light yellowing that can occur with a superficial petechial reaction. These tissues were worked very hard, and this amount of bruising would place a significant amount of metabolic stress onto the tissues involved, which would never be an intended outcome. When the goal is to just "work into" tissues rather than truly engage with them whilst approaching an individual with considered rationale, then bruising occurs.

Ultimately, bruising does not occur instantaneously or without warning. There will be a build-up, and being aware of how the tissues you are working on react is very important for that. Indiscriminate technique or the belief that the purpose of IASTM is to work harder and more deeply into the tissues will result in bruising. But that is your decision as a practitioner, not the fault of the technique. If you are bruising people on a regular basis or without intending to, you are using this technique wrongly and it is resulting in tissues being overtreated.

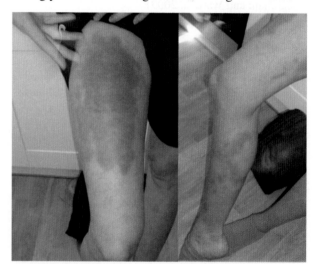

Figure A.1: Extensive bruising caused by excessive force being used by practitioners who have been taught to "get into" tissues

Research

The most commonly quoted research for IASTM is that undertaken by Terry Loghmani (Loghmani and Warden, 2009), wherein rat medial collateral ligaments (MCLs) were resected then repaired bilaterally, one side treated and one side not. At seven days after the operation, instrument-assisted cross-friction massage was used on one MCL for one minute, three times a week for three weeks. Ligaments treated with IASTM were found to be thirty-one percent stronger and thirty-four percent stiffer than untreated ligaments. The implications, extrapolated for humans from these results in rats, are that in the two–twelve-week stages of healing, significant improvements could be made in the tissues' ability to accept and tolerate load (see Figure A.2).

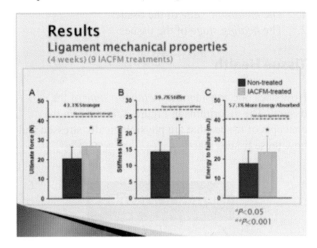

Figure A.2: Ligament mechanical properties (four weeks; nine IASTM treatments)

This may be explained by the cellular and global structural changes that were also noted on the ligaments. As the research states, "The scar region of IASTM-treated ligaments at four weeks post injury also appeared to have greater cellularity, with collagen fiber bundles appearing to be oriented more along the longitudinal axis of the ligament than observed in contralateral non-treated ligaments" (see Figure A.3).

The images of the changes in the cellular activity of the treated tissues are quite remarkable and, if taken directly into the context of human healing, the potential gains which could be achieved are certainly significant. Moreover, the subjects (rats) did not undertake any physical rehabilitation as a human subject under treatment would. One could speculate that had the rats undergone appropriate loading exercises, the gains they made would have been significantly greater still.

Additional work has been undertaken by Gehlsen et al. (1999), looking into the differing effects of utilizing IASTM at different pressures, which found that increased pressures resulted in increased fibroblastic activity.

If translated to the clinical situation, this could influence how much pressure was utilized. The clinician could consider how much activity was likely to be present on a cellular level at the time of treatment, and which reaction it would be appropriate to induce. Deeper tissue work would potentially result in an increase in cellular activity that may aggravate the tissues if already inflammatory, or reinitiate healing in chronically scarred tissue.

Davidson et al. (1997) discovered increased fibroblast proliferation in the IASTM group of their study: "the study suggests that IASTM may promote healing via increased fibroblast recruitment."

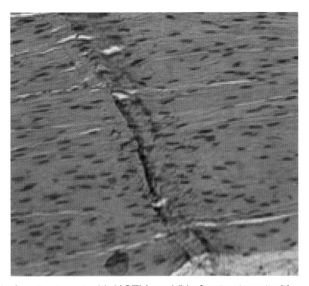

Figure A.3: Images of the changes in the cellular activity: (a) before treatment with IASTM, and (b) after treatment with IASTM

The majority of published work on IASTM is on cellular-level studies in rat subjects. The remainder is predominantly case studies. Kinnective wanted to look at the clinical effects that IASTM may achieve, and therefore undertook some pilot studies that are not yet published but show some interesting results. The study design was based on clinical effects that had been seen in practice. The first was an investigation into the effects of the Kinnective technique: an IASTM on hamstring length. Results were that the mean percentage increase in length in the test group was 49.66% compared with 11.44% in the control group. The second pilot looked into the effects of IASTM on the electromyographic activity of the hamstring muscle. Interestingly, comparison with the control group suggested that IASTM increased electromyographic activity in the hamstring.

How Does IASTM Work?

Theoretically, the rationale, indications, and contraindications for use of IASTM are the same as those of manual soft-tissue treatment. However, a well designed stainless steel instrument produces increased sensation, delivering more information from the tissues than is felt with hands alone. It also allows for greater depth and specificity and quicker and more effective release with motion. If you like to work with functional movement patterns or treating under motion, this is a perfect technique to work with.

Considerations for IASTM Use

What Are You Trying to Achieve?

What is the objective of treatment, i.e. how is the tissue potentially being impacted? Considering globally what can be achieved with soft tissues, you could have five categories of beneficial effect:

1. Improvement in sliding and gliding
2. Breakdown of adhesions and restrictions
3. Increase in cellular activity
4. Activation/facilitation of muscle
5. Deactivation/inhibition of muscle.

These will be considered the *clinical objectives*. They will determine the type of stroke undertaken and the edge of the instrument used, and, as discussed earlier, the pressure induced on the tissues.

After selecting one of these five options, next consider it within the context of the *clinical goals*:

1. Reduction in pain
2. Increase in ROM
3. Reduction in sensitivity
4. Reduction of muscle spasm
5. Facilitation of muscle activity.

This will also impact on the clinical decision making regarding the stroke, speed, depth of pressure, and contact surface utilized.

In addition to this, be aware of *clinical considerations*, which determine the application of the decided technique. One of the most significant clinical considerations is the *tissue health*, and there are two main determining factors to consider here when using IASTM:

1. The *metabolic state* of the tissues
2. The *healing stage* of the tissues.

Tissue Health

How does one consider the *metabolic state* of the tissues? The algorithms in Figure A.4 underpin the concepts of tissues that are physiologically stressed and how these tissues react.

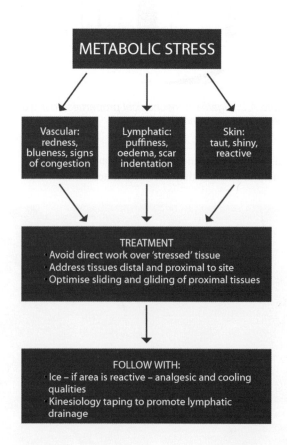

METABOLIC STRESS

| Vascular: redness, blueness, signs of congestion | Lymphatic: puffiness, oedema, scar indentation | Skin: taut, shiny, reactive |

TREATMENT
· Avoid direct work over 'stressed' tissue
· Address tissues distal and proximal to site
· Optimise sliding and gliding of proximal tissues

FOLLOW WITH:
· Ice – if area is reactive – analgesic and cooling qualities
· Kinesiology taping to promote lymphatic drainage

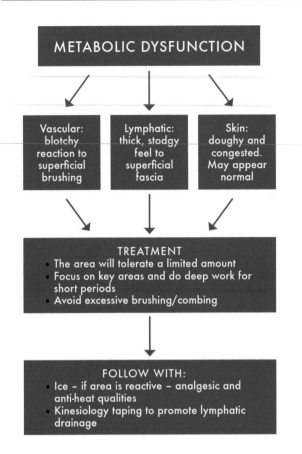

METABOLIC DYSFUNCTION

- **Vascular:** blotchy reaction to superficial brushing
- **Lymphatic:** thick, stodgy feel to superficial fascia
- **Skin:** doughy and congested. May appear normal

TREATMENT
- The area will tolerate a limited amount
- Focus on key areas and do deep work for short periods
- Avoid excessive brushing/combing

FOLLOW WITH:
- Ice – if area is reactive – analgesic and anti-heat qualities
- Kinesiology taping to promote lymphatic drainage

Figure A.4: The algorithms underpinning the concepts of tissues that are physiologically stressed and how these tissues react

These tissues require an altered approach with IASTM in particular, as they are more prone to being reactive, both in a subjective symptomatic way, i.e. with soreness and sensitivity, and also objectively, i.e. with bruising or redness.

Consider a clinical objective of improving sliding and gliding with the clinical goal of increasing ROM. This would be undertaken usually with a larger contact surface, using swift, longer strokes of a shallower depth. Adding movement to the tissues whilst applying the technique would assist in the gliding and sliding of the tissues. If you were concerned about tissues being under metabolic stress, for example in an acute phase, then you would work at tissues distal and proximal to the involved site to avoid overstressing tissues. Whereas if you were undertaking this task on an individual with good metabolic tissue health undergoing optimization, you would work directly over the area involved under a functional loading pattern.

Therefore, the treatment undertaken is a combination of the chosen clinical objective to achieve the clinical goal within the clinical considerations, particularly considering tissue health. Different techniques can be utilized to achieve different effects, some of which will be discussed later in this appendix.

With any manual technique, suiting it to the individual is an inherent part of the "art" of the practice, and IASTM is no different in this respect. This is cultivated with good initial technique combined with experience.

In the descriptions of the techniques contained within this book, please refer to the image in Figure A.5 to orient yourself with the clinical edges of the Kinnective instrument. There is a "correct" orientation of the instrument on the skin, which produces the best feel and feedback. The various strokes and holds of the instrument and how to use them in the correct orientation are confusing to write. If you would like further information on this, please refer to the video on the Kinnective website called Basic Instrument Use, in which this is covered.

Personal note: *Whilst I appreciate that many therapists use IASTM for almost everything, I use it as an adjunct to my soft-tissue techniques and only when I feel it's needed. In my opinion, IASTM comes into its own when working pre-event as a whole-body treatment (leading to the sensation of lightness and spring, according to the athletes I treat), and around joints and difficult-to-reach places.*

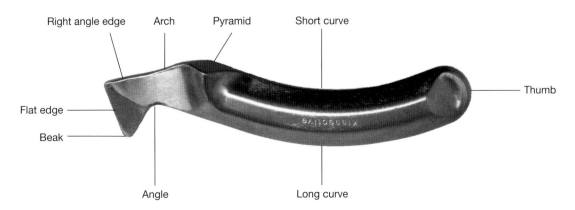

Right angle edge   Arch   Pyramid   Short curve

Flat edge

Beak

Thumb

Angle

Long curve

Figure A.5: The Kinnective instrument

References

Davidson CJ, Ganion LR, Gehlsen GM, Verhoestra B, Roepke JE, and Sevier TL (1997) Rat tendon morphologic and functional changes resulting from soft tissue mobilization. *Medicine and Science in Sports and Exercise* 29(3): 313–319

Gehlsen GM, Ganion LR, and Helfst R (1999) Fibroblast responses to variation in soft tissue mobilization pressure. *Medicine and Science in Sports and Exercise* 31(4): 531–535

Loghmani MT and Warden SJ (2009) Instrument-assisted cross-fiber massage accelerates knee ligament healing. *Journal of Orthopaedic and Sports Physical Therapy* 39(7): 506–514; doi: 10.2519/jospt.2009.2997

Nielsen A (1995) Gua Sha: *Traditional Technique for Modern Practice*. Edinburgh: Churchill Livingstone

Stillerman E (2009) *Modalities for Massage and Bodywork*. Edinburgh: Mosby Elsevier. pp. 115–126

Index